Good Food, Good Medicine

Advice on nutrition and lifestyle for good health

Dr John Pembrey

*To Bill and Dorothy,
with very best wishes
John Pembrey*

First Edition - 2008

Published by **Imprimata**

A CIP Catalogue record for this book is available
from the British Library

ISBN 978-1-906192-11-2

Printed and bound by CPI Antony Rowe, Eastbourne

Imprimata

Imprimata Publishers Limited
50 Albemarle Street, London W1S 4BD.

Dedications

To help improve the quality of life of everyone from every country and whatever religious and political views. We may disagree but we can still help each other.

I would like to thank my wife Julie and children Mark, Graham, Alexander and Anna for tolerating me while spending a lot of thought and time on writing this book. With thanks to Iain Burns, Mark Bracey and all at Imprimata for making this book possible and to Ian and Marjory Chapman for their support.

To the readers: I hope you find the book helpful. Any feedback, including criticism, is welcome so that any mistakes or misinformation can be corrected.

I would like to thank the nutritional pioneers and many authors for providing the information contained in this book.

Mention should be made of Hippocrates the famous and wise Greek physician who in about 450 B.C. was quoted as saying "Let food be your medicine and medicine be your food." This quote inspired the title of this book.

I would like to remember my grandfather, Marcus Seymour Pembrey (1868–1934), a physiologist who also recognised the importance of diet.

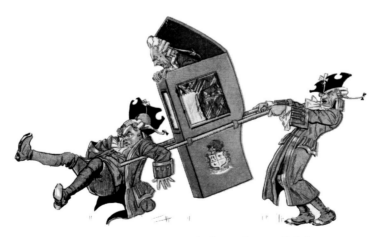

The human or horse works best when well-fed,
And feeds best when well worked.
Professor Pembrey, F.R.S.

Contents

Introduction

Working as a General Practitioner of medicine for over thirty years has made me realise that the number of people suffering from many medical problems could be decreased by an improvement in lifestyle and nutrition. These medical problems include cardiovascular disease, mental health problems, osteoporosis and cancer.

Medication can be effective and is sometimes essential and lifesaving. However it is often ineffective and expensive with a risk of side effects.

Many elderly patients take a confusing amount of medication, which frequently causes side effects. If some medication could be stopped or reduced this would be helpful.

I am convinced that if the general public were better informed about lifestyle and nutrition they would have less medical problems, less investigations, less operations and less medication. Public demand is a powerful force in promoting changes in such things as choice of food, drink and other lifestyle factors. This book is an attempt to inform people about how to improve their nutrition and lifestyle.

There is still a great deal that we do not know about nutrition and a lot more research is required. However a great deal of research has already been carried out and we have acquired a large amount of knowledge on the subject. This knowledge would be of more benefit if it were passed on to a larger amount of people and put into practice

"A little knowledge that acts is worth infinitely more than much knowledge that is idle"

Kahlil Gibran. Poet

Diet and population studies comparing eastern and western diets show that diet has a huge impact on our health. People on the Greek island of Crete and in China who ate a diet that had developed over thousands of years had far less chronic illness than those on a more 'modern' diet in western countries. Their incidence of cardiovascular disease, diabetes, asthma, osteoporosis, osteoarthritis, depression, other mental health problems, dementia and cancer were far less than in the western world and they had a longer life. The western world has this information but is largely ignoring it. It is spending an increasing amount on doctors, expensive diagnostic equipment and treatment.

An increasing amount is also being spent on new drugs and research. Side effects of drugs are a major problem and very costly. Doctors are under increasing pressure to monitor and treat chronic conditions which could have been prevented. These self-induced preventable illnesses are causing a huge amount of disability, suffering, work loss, financial loss and social cost.

Research suggests that the best diets such as the Mediterranean, Japanese and Chinese are mainly vegetarian but with fish and a small amount of meat.

- The fish are wild and not farmed.
- The small amount of meat is from small grass fed animals such as sheep, goats or chickens. Very little or no beef is eaten.
- Cheese is made from goats and sheep's milk rather than cow's milk. Very little cow's milk, cheese or butter is consumed.
- Bread is wholemeal.
- Very little refined sugar and processed food is eaten.
- A small regular intake of alcohol is common and usually in the form of wine rather than beer or spirits.

Health is better in the rural areas of these countries. This may be because of less smoking and pollution. There is also fresher produce and less temptation from processed fast food. Another factor is that people and families with medical problems tend to move closer to hospitals and doctors.

The Seven Countries Study

This was a very important study of the effect of different diets on health. It can never be repeated as most of the countries are now moving towards an unhealthy western diet.

The study started in 1958. The team was led by an American doctor, Anzel Keys. 12,763 healthy men between the ages of 40 and 59, from seven different countries were studied. The main interest was in coronary heart disease as the number of people having heart attacks had increased dramatically in the West.

The study showed that the people in Crete had far less heart attacks than those in Holland and the USA. It is since this study that the Mediterranean diet has been strongly recommended.

Crete had by far the lowest coronary mortality of the countries studied, yet serum cholesterol levels were average (5.2) and not as low as Yugoslavia (4.5) or Japan (3.9). In general cholesterol levels rose according to the saturated fat intake which is mainly from animal meat and dairy products.

A French professor Serge Renaud on seeing the results in 1980 concluded that " Something protects Cretans which does not reduce their cholesterol"

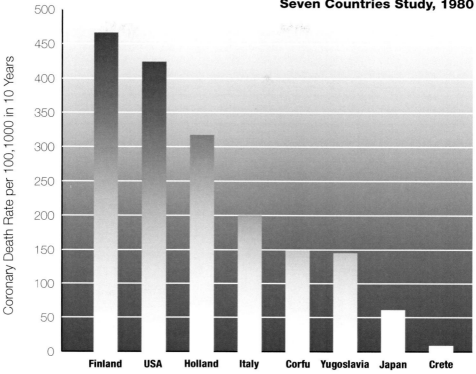

**Death from Coronary Heart Disease over 10 Years
Seven Countries Study, 1980**

Coronary Death Rate per 100,1000 in 10 Years

Finland　USA　Holland　Italy　Corfu　Yugoslavia　Japan　Crete

Cholesterol levels - Seven Countries Study 1980

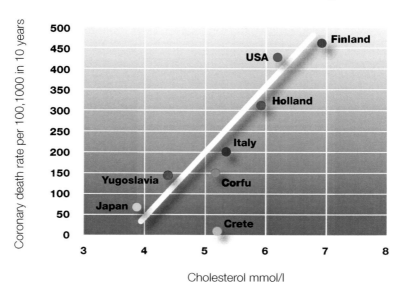

Coronary death rate per 100,1000 in 10 years

Cholesterol mmol/l

Diets compared 1987

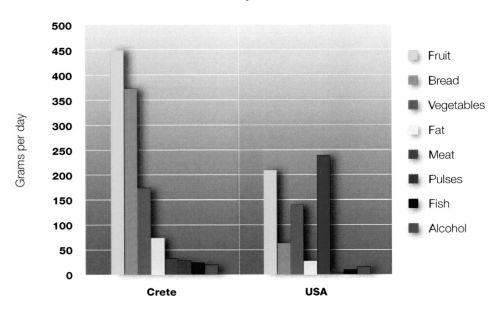

Nutritional Habits per area (grams per day)			
	Crete	Holland	U.S.A.
Fruit	464	82	233
Bread	390	252	97
Vegetables	191	117	171
Fat	95	79	33
Meat	35	138	273
Pulses	30	2	1
Fish	18	12	3
Alcohol	15	3	6

and guessed that the difference in diets was the much greater intake of alpha-linolenic acid (a precursor of omega-3) in the Cretan diet.

Surprisingly Crete had a higher fat intake than other countries but this was mainly in the form of olive oil and other plant fats rather than the high intake of saturated fat from meat and dairy products in Western countries. The meat intake in Crete was less than in any other country and this was mainly from smaller animals such as chickens, sheep and goats rather than cattle.

Characteristics of the Mediterranean diet:

- High ratio of monounsaturated (olive oil) to saturated fats.
- High consumption of vegetables especially Greens.
- High consumption of fruit.
- High consumption of cereals especially wholegrain bread.
- High consumption of herbs.
- Moderate consumption of fish.
- Moderate consumption of nuts.
- Low consumption of meat and sugar.
- Low consumption of milk and dairy products.
- Moderate consumption of alcohol.

Japan had the second best figures for heart attacks and by far the lowest fat intake:

As percentage of calorie intake	Japan	Crete
Total Fat	10%	40%
Saturated fat	3%	8%
Polyunsaturated fat	4%	4%
Monounsaturated fat	3%	28%
Cholesterol levels	3.9%	5.2%

In overall mortality Japan was second worst while Crete was still the best. At that time, hypertension (high blood pressure) was common in Japan because of the high salt intake and haemorrhagic strokes were common. The very low fat intakes and cholesterol levels were thought to aggravate the problem by supplying inadequate fat in the brain to help support the blood vessels.

The men from Finland had an active lifestyle but consumed a great deal of saturated fat from red meat and dairy products. The fish was often salty. Only a small amount of fresh fruit and vegetables were consumed and these often came from selenium deficient soil. Their cholesterol levels tended to be high (over 7.0). In 1991, thirty three years after the beginning of the study 50% of the 700 Cretan men were alive whereas *none of the men from Finland had survived.*

Overall Mortality over 10 Years - Seven Countries Study, 1980

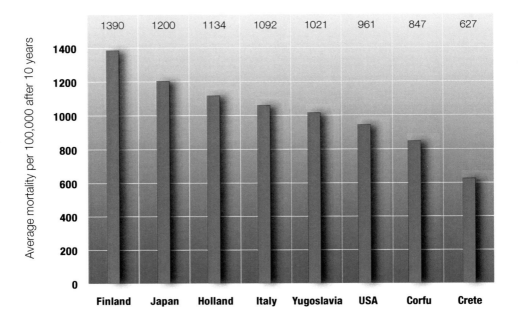

Since 1980 Japan has made efforts to increase its fat intake

	1958	1999
Fat intake as % of calories	10	20
Average cholesterol levels mmol/l	3.9	4.9
The coronary heart death rate per 100,000	60	35
The stroke death rate per 100,000	1100	250

A higher consumption of animal fat and cholesterol was associated with reduced risk of stroke.

These studies suggest that although high cholesterol increases the risk of a thrombotic (ischaemic) stroke, low cholesterol increases the risk of a haemorrhagic stroke.

Salt intake and hypertension were also reduced.

Japan became the country with the highest life expectancy. Surprisingly the heart attack rate did not increase with the increase of fat and cholesterol. This suggests that we require a certain amount of fat in our diet and that a very low, as well as a high, cholesterol level may cause ill health.

Since 1980 Finland has made efforts to reduce its saturated fat intake. There have also been campaigns to reduce salt intake and smoking. Selenium is now added to the soil and more vegetables are eaten.

General

Vegetable and fruit whole foods in their natural state contain small amounts of numerous vitamins, minerals and phytonutrients which are important for our health. They contain fibre which helps prevent constipation and other bowel problems. The fibre slows the absorption of sugars, protein and fat which reduces the risk of cardiovascular disease, diabetes and mental health problems.

The seeds of the plants provide very important essential fatty acids omega-3 and omega-6. These are required to make prostaglandins which are hormone like substances that control the physiology of our body. For example they control inflammation, nerve transmission, blood clotting and muscle contraction. They have an important effect on the risk of thrombosis, hypertension, chronic inflammation and mental health disorders. The optimum diets have the correct amount of Omega-3 in proportion to Omega-6, which reduces inflammation and the risk of thrombosis. Both Omega-3 and Omega-6 are present in all plants, seeds and nuts, but the amounts of each vary. Omega-3 is associated with chlorophyll which is the green pigment in plant leaves and algae.

Green algae are at the bottom of the food chain for all fish. The herbivores and very small fish eat the algae. The carnivorous fish eat the smaller fish.

Green plants are at the bottom of the food chain for all animals. The large vegetarian herbivores such as deer and cows eat the plants. Carnivorous animals eat the herbivores.

A certain amount of saturated fat and monounsaturated fat as well as the polyunsaturated Omega-3 and Omega-6 is required for good health. Saturated fat tends to increase cholesterol but cholesterol is important for health and although high blood cholesterol levels increase your risk of heart disease low cholesterol levels appear to increase your risk of mental health problems and possibly stroke and cancer.

The optimum cholesterol level seems to be about 5mmol/l

Compared with the optimum diets for good health, the western diet has a lack of fresh whole food fruit and vegetables. This is usually due to choice rather than availability. Because of this we tend to lack important nutrients which would help protect us from such illnesses as heart attacks, strokes, diabetes and cancer.

We have too much meat, dairy produce and eggs. These provide too much saturated fat and protein. They also provide an excess of hormones which may increase our risk of certain cancers.

We have too much refined bread and sugar. This provides calories, but very little in the way of nutrients. The risk of obesity and diabetes is increased.

We have too much processed and refined foods which often contain an excess of sugar or salt as a preservative as well as other additives. They provide calories and taste nice but provide very few nutrients and often contain trans-fats which damage our health.

It is very important to realise that diet is a delicate balance between avoiding deficiency and avoiding excess. Some things that it is recommended we avoid can be taken in small amounts without harm, and those that are recommended should not be taken in excess as this may cause harm.

"Everything in moderation" is good advice and the following quotation is one of the most important in medicine and life:

> *"All things are poisons and there is nothing that is harmless, the dose alone decides that something is not poison."*
>
> **Paracelsus. 16th century Swiss physician and father of toxicology.**

There follows a more in depth study of nutrition and lifestyle. I have tried to keep it simple.

> *"Simplicity is the ultimate sophistication."*
>
> **Leonardo da Vinci.**

Dr John Pembrey, 2007

Avoid too much salt

History of Salt

When many millions of years ago man was roaming the plains of Africa there was very little salt available. Food contained more potassium than sodium and did not contain much chloride. The body's kidneys adapted to conserve sodium and chloride.

Over the next four million years salt remained scarce. In Roman times it was so precious that it was used as money in trading. It is only over the last 500 years that salt has become easily available and cheap.

Salt was found to prevent bacterial growth and was therefore used to preserve food that was stored or transported great distances. It was used in canned food to prevent food poisoning especially botulism. People became used to the salt in their food and now find non-salted food very bland.

Unfortunately a high salt intake raises blood pressure. Because of genetic variation some people have adapted faster than others and can tolerate salt without raising their blood pressure when young. However this adaptation often reduces with age.

How excess salt causes Hypertension

If too much salt is in the diet the kidneys excrete more sodium in the urine. If the excretion rate is not sufficient the arteries constrict to raise the blood pressure and force more sodium through the semi-permeable membranes of the kidney. The constricted arteries retain fluid in order to dilute the excess of sodium in the extra cellular fluid. If the sodium excess continues the blood volume increases and the vascular system adapts by keeping the blood pressure raised.

There are a few isolated communities in which hypertension is not seen, such as the Yanomamo Indians (Amazon), Kalahari Bushmen (Botswana), and remote Pacific islanders. These people have very low salt intakes of 2g or less.

- The physiological requirement for salt is less than 1g per day.
- The recommended intake is 1.2 g (500 mg sodium)
- The recommended maximum intake is 6g daily.
- The average adult intake in the UK is 10 to 12 g daily. Hypertension occurs in 15% of UK adults.
- Diet is a greater causative factor in hypertension than genes.
- In South Japan average salt intake is about 17g daily. Hypertension occurs in over 20% of adults.
- In Northern Japan average salt intake is about 25g daily. Hypertension occurs in over 35% of adults

Salt and Hypertension

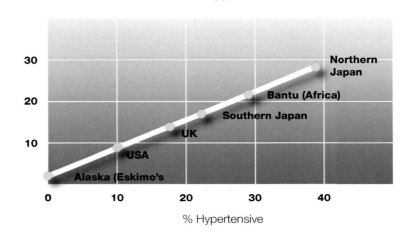

Modified from ABC of Nutrition. BMJ 1985.

Hypertension, the size of the problem

It is estimated that 20% of adults in the Western world have high blood pressure. That is about 7 million people in the UK aged over 25 years. The incidence rises with age and by 60 years of age over 60% are affected.

For many years Life Insurance companies have known that a raised blood pressure reduces life expectancy. People with a diastolic blood pressure above 100 have twice the normal death rate for their age.

Hypertension increases the risk of strokes and dementia. It increases the risk of heart disease, in particular cardiac failure. It also increases the risk of kidney failure and poor eyesight.

Blood pressure

Normal blood pressure is about 140/85 or less. High is over 160/90. The systolic pressure (the first number) is the pressure created by the heart ventricles contracting and forcing blood into the arteries. The diastolic pressure (the second number) is that which remains in the arteries when the heart is relaxed.

About 10% of cases of hypertension are related to other medical problems such as kidney disease, adrenal tumours and renal artery stenosis. The other 90% is called 'essential hypertension' and the main cause is almost certainly a chronic high salt intake as well as other nutritional factors.

Blood pressure depends on the strength of the pump (the heart) and the resistance in the peripheral arterial circulation. The resistance is affected by the viscosity or "stickiness" of the blood and the elasticity and diameter of the arteries and arterioles. It follows that reducing the stickiness of the blood and dilating the arteries will reduce resistance and blood pressure.

How to make the blood less sticky and reduce blood pressure

Making the blood less sticky reduces peripheral resistance and reduces blood pressure. It also reduces the risk of thrombosis. Thrombosis may cause a stroke, heart attack, deep vein leg thrombosis or pulmonary embolus.

Omega-3 foods reduce the clotting time of blood – Omega-3 can be obtained from oily fish such as mackerel, herring, sardines, salmon, tuna and trout or from vegetarian sources flax, hemp seeds, walnuts and their oils, mustard seeds, pumpkin seeds and leafy green vegetables.

Although Omega-3 and Omega-6 fatty acids are both essential the balance is important. An excess of Omega-6 relative to Omega-3 can increase the risk of thrombosis.

Certain **fruit and vegetables**, particularly tomatoes but also strawberries, grapefruit and melons, contain a component, named P3 that reduces platelet activity and the risk of thrombosis.

Garlic reduces blood platelet stickiness as well as cholesterol.

Turmeric a yellow spice in Indian food reduces platelet stickiness and relaxes arteries.

Vitamin C in fruit and vegetables also reduces blood stickiness and improves the health of the arteries.

How to dilate the arteries and reduce blood pressure

Blood pressure is determined partly by the balance of certain minerals in the muscle cells of the arterial wall which cause either constriction or relaxation. The amount of constriction and relaxation of the artery wall decreases with age as the elastic fibres in the wall become less efficient and calcification and atheroma occur. Constriction of the artery walls raises the blood pressure and relaxation of the artery walls reduces blood pressure.

A higher **sodium** and **lower potassium** than normal inside the muscle cell causes contraction of the muscles and constriction of the artery. The higher the sodium relative to potassium, the higher the blood pressure.

A **higher calcium** and **lower magnesium** than normal inside the muscle cell causes contraction of the muscles and constriction of the artery. The higher the calcium relative to magnesium the higher the blood pressure.

A high calcium low magnesium diet raises blood pressure.

Because of our high dairy diet we usually have a high calcium intake but are often deficient in magnesium. Cow's milk contains a higher ratio of calcium to magnesium than the 2 parts of calcium to 1 of magnesium which is ideal for humans (Milk 10 to 1 . Cheese 25 to 1)

The refining of bread and sugar removes the calcium and magnesium. Calcium is then added to white bread by law but not magnesium.

Magnesium can be obtained from wholegrain cereals and bread, brown rice, nuts, seeds and beans. It is also present in pulses (beans and peas) and green leaf plants.

Between 1972 and 1992 the Finns switched from table salt to a mixed potassium and magnesium salt. (Pan Salt)

- The National average blood pressure fell dramatically.
- Heart attacks were reduced by 55% (men) 68% (women)
- Strokes were reduced by 62%

Sodium/potassium ratio

In animals in general there is a ratio of three times the amount of potassium compared to sodium.

In plants there is a ratio of about twenty times the amount of potassium compared to sodium as they have no nervous system and do not need to transmit nerve impulses.

Sodium increases blood pressure. Potassium lowers blood pressure.

In populations who have three times more potassium than sodium in their diet hypertension is virtually unknown and does not occur with advancing age.

The ideal amount of dietary sodium should be three times less than the amount of potassium. This ratio is only possible by eating natural foods and avoiding processed foods.

Due to softening processes tap water contains more sodium than potassium. Calcium and magnesium are largely removed.

Most processed food is high in salt and low in potassium:

	(mg/100g)	
	Sodium	Potassium
Cornflakes	1160	99
Canned luncheon meat	1050	140
Canned frankfurter	980	98
Fruit pie	210	120
Cheddar cheese	268	31

Most natural foods such as fruit and vegetables and even meats are low in salt and high in potassium:

	(mg/100ml)	
	Sodium	Potassium
Steak (grilled)	56	390
Apple	2	120
Avocado	2	400
Corn	1	280
Cows milk	161	410

Foods high in Salt

Foods high in salt are always processed foods:

Bread – an average 40g slice contains 0.5g salt. Four slices contain 2g.
Advice: salt intake can be reduced by choosing low salt bread or making
your own bread in an automatic bread maker.

Cereals – vary in salt content. Cornflakes have 1g per bowl.
Advice. Look for low salt, low sugar cereals.

Soups – most ready prepared canned or powdered soups are high in salt.
A large cup (200mls) of soup contains from 2 to 5 g of salt.
Advice. Look for low salt or make own fresh soup.

Processed meat - such as sausages, bacon and ham are high in salt .
One sausage usually contains over 1g of salt.
Advice: avoid – they are also high in saturated fat.

Ready meals and pizzas - often contain over 3g of salt in a serving.
Advice: avoid or limit amount.

Comment

*"Salt, in the amount that is eaten in the UK, is a chronic long-term toxin
which slowly raises blood pressure from childhood onwards so that, as
people reach middle and old age, they are put at ever increasing risk of
death and disability through strokes, heart attacks and heart failure that
raised blood pressure causes".*

"If reducing salt intake to below 6g a day is successful, it will result in the biggest improvement in public health since the introduction of clean water and drains in the 19th century."

Professor Graham MacGregor

Professor of Cardiovascular Medicine, St George's Hospital,London.
Chairman of the Blood Pressure Association
Chairman of Consensus Action on Salt and Health.

Dietary and lifestyle Hypertension treatment.

- Reduce sodium intake by reducing salt.
- Avoid an excess of processed foods (contain hidden salt)
- Avoid excess saturated fat.(Increases blood stickiness)
- Have adequate essential fatty acids (Omega-3 reduces blood viscosity.)
- Avoid excess sugar (this stimulates insulin to retain salt.)
- Avoid excess of coffee and tea.
- Avoid excess alcohol.
- Avoid excess weight.
- Increase exercise.
- Avoid smoking (which constricts arteries).
- Avoid stress (raises cortisol and adrenalin)
- Increase magnesium, calcium, potassium and fibre intake all of which reduce blood pressure by having adequate fruit, vegetables, wholemeal bread, brown rice, soybeans, nuts and seeds. Eating just two bananas a day can lower blood pressure by 10%.
- Eat a Mediterranean type diet with fresh tomatoes, garlic, oily fish, olive oil and red wine. These all improve the health of the arteries.

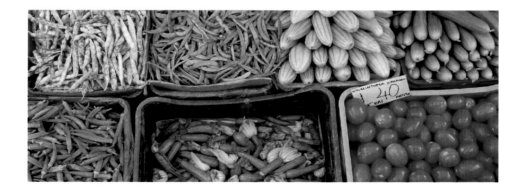

Avoid too much Meat and Dairy products.

Protein

We need a constant supply of protein which is not stored in the body like fat. It is required to make muscle, organs such as the heart, skin, hair and enzymes. Together with essential fatty acids the essential amino acids provided by protein synthesise the important neurotransmitters serotonin, adrenalin, noradrenalin, dopamine and acetylcholine that are essential for our mental health.

A variety of vegetable protein is usually required to supply all the eight essential amino acids. The body is able to produce twelve amino acids from other compounds in the body and these are labelled as non-essential. Soya beans contain most of the essential amino acids but are low in one, methionine. Meat, fish, milk and eggs contain all the essential amino acids.

Most people in the western world have too much protein. As well as protein in vegetables they have a large amount of animal protein in meat, poultry, eggs, milk, cheese and other dairy products.

Recommended protein intake is 45g daily for women and 55g daily for men.

The average US protein intake is 65g daily for women and 90g daily for men.

3 oz of any meat contains about 25g of protein. A cup of lentil soup contains 8g. An egg contains 6g. Almond nuts 6g. A slice of whole wheat bread 3g.

In the Mediterranean diet meat is only eaten about once a week.

High Protein Diet

A high protein diet increases the risk of **osteoporosis**. The breakdown of proteins and amino acids makes the blood more acidic. This causes calcium to be taken from the bones to counteract the acidity.

A high protein diet increases the risk of **kidney stones**. The breakdown of protein and increased acidity increases the excretion of calcium oxalate in the urine and makes it more likely to crystallize and form stones.

A high protein diet increases the risk of **gout**. The breakdown of protein produces purines . The breakdown of purine nucleic acids produce uric acid which increases the risk of gout, especially in those who lack an enzyme which helps the breakdown of uric acid.

A high protein diet increases the risk of **atherosclerosis.** Excessive protein increases homocysteine levels which increases the risk of atherosclerosis (furring up of arteries). This makes heart attacks and strokes more likely.

A high protein diet creates an excess of arachidonic acid and the **inflammatory** prostaglandin 2. This increases the risk of atherosclerosis, **osteoarthritis and cancer.**

Protein and Osteoporosis

A protein rich diet is acid forming (mainly due to the breakdown of sulphur-containing amino acids). The acid is counteracted in the body by alkaline agent's potassium and calcium. When the body's reserves of potassium are used up calcium is taken from the bones and excreted.

A high protein diet therefore causes calcium deficiency. This increases the risk of osteoporosis. The incidence of osteoporosis induced fractures of the hip and vertebrae in the spine have greatly increased over the last fifty years and this is thought to be partly due to our increased intake of protein in particular meat, milk, cheese and eggs.

Meat and milk in excess or together with vitamin and cod-liver oil supplements may also provide too much vitamin A which also aggravates osteoporosis

African Bantu's have a low protein, low fat and low calcium diet but virtually no osteoporosis. They have a lot of fruit, nuts and vegetables and plenty of vitamin D inducing sunshine.

Eskimos have a high protein, high fat and high calcium diet and have an exceptionally high incidence of osteoporosis. They have very little fruit, nuts and vegetables and very little sunshine.

Herbivores and Carnivores

We tend to think of ourselves as omnivores, but our dentition and digestive systems suggest that we are designed to be mainly herbivores and may not be able to cope with more than a small amount of meat.

Humans and Herbivores	Carnivores and omnivores
*Small mouth relative to skull size.	*Large mouth relative to skull size.
*Flexible jaw and well developed facial muscles for chewing.	*Inflexible jaw and poorly developed facial muscles for holding food.
*Blunt short teeth for chewing.	*Sharp long teeth for tearing and holding.
*Saliva with carbohydrate digesting enzymes.	*Saliva with no digesting enzymes.
*Simple or multiple chamber stomach.	*Simple large stomach
*Stomach less than 30% of total digestive tract volume.	*Stomach over 60% of total digestive tract volume.
*pH of stomach 4 to 5.	*pH of stomach 1 or less.
*Small intestine over ten times body length.	*Small intestine about five times body length.
*Colon long and sacculated.	*Colon short and smooth.
*Liver cannot detoxify Vit. A.	*Liver can detoxify Vit. A.
*Concentrated urine.	*Very concentrated urine.
*Flat nails or blunt hooves.	*Sharp claws.

Adapted from Herbivore, omnivore or carnivore? Milton R. Mills

The pH of our blood is slightly alkaline and has to be maintained within a narrow range from 7.35 to 7.45. The body regulates this by excreting excess acid or alkali in the urine or increasing or decreasing the excretion of carbonic acid (carbon dioxide in water) via the lungs.

Herbivores, which eat only plants, have an alkaline urine. The plant 'acids' such as citric, malic, benzoic, tartaric and oxalic are in fact alkali-forming. Lactic acid is also alkali-forming.

Carnivores eating only animal meat have an acid urine. Meat protein is high in sulphur which the body converts to sulphuric acid before excretion in the urine. Meat is also high in phosphorus which the body converts to phosphoric acid before excretion in the urine.

Some humans such as the Eskimo, American Indians and the Masai tribe in Africa have adapted to a high animal or fish diet over thousands of years. The enzymes that help metabolise plants are reduced whereas the enzymes that metabolise meat have increased.

Any sudden change of this longstanding diet is detrimental to their health. For instance the American Indians were put in reservations and given benefits so that they no longer needed to hunt for buffalo or work hard. Changing from a high protein diet to a high carbohydrate, high sugar, high fat diet together with a lack of exercise caused a high incidence of depression, obesity, diabetes and cardiovascular disease.

Milk and Osteoporosis

For many years we have been persuaded that we need cow's milk and its products to obtain enough calcium for our bones.

But why does the cow not get osteoporosis? It is a large animal with large bones. It has a calf every year and produces large amounts of milk with a high calcium and protein content. Where does it get all the required replacement calcium and protein? In the natural state it is purely from eating green leafy plants.

No animal meat. No milk or cheese. No eggs.

The calf is weaned off its mother's milk after a few months and then relies on a vegetarian diet and water to maintain its large bones and musculature.

The largest land animals have always been vegetarian herbivores, from dinosaurs to the present day elephants, giraffes and rhinos.

Amongst the wild animals there is very little record of the common western medical problems such as cardiovascular disease, diabetes, osteoporosis and cancer.

It is the domesticated animals such as cows, horses and dogs who are often fed incorrect diets that suffer from an excess of infections, nutritional deficiencies and cancer.

Carnivorous animals also avoid osteoporosis by eating wild animals that have fed on green leafy plants or eat fish that have fed on green algae.

It appears that all the mammals do well if they live in harmony with their genetic makeup and natural foods.

Calcium balance

Fruit and vegetables supply calcium efficiently together with beneficial vitamin A (carotenoids), vitamin C, vitamin K, magnesium, numerous phytonutrients and minimal saturated fat. They are high in potassium relative to protein and alkaline which reduces calcium loss from the bones.

Milk supplies plenty of calcium but the high protein content causes increased excretion of calcium. This means that someone on a high protein diet requires about 800 mg of calcium a day whereas a vegetarian can get by on 200 mg. Dairy produce also has very low levels of magnesium and high levels of vitamin A which may also increase the risk of osteoporosis.

Magnesium, potassium and vitamin D aid the absorption of calcium.

Sodium and high protein decrease absorption.

The worst foods for calcium balance are those high in protein but low in calcium such as meat, fish and eggs. They cause a negative balance by causing increased excretion of calcium. For example 100g of meat will cause the loss of about 20mg of calcium from the body whereas 100g of spring greens will contribute about 20mg of calcium.

Dairy foods are high in protein as well as calcium and so increase calcium loss as well as providing calcium. They are beneficial at normal absorption but become a very inefficient source of calcium if absorption is reduced as is common in old age.

Cheddar cheese contains about 720mg of calcium per 100g. Because of the protein content it only contributes 38mg (5%) to calcium balance at normal absorption and only 11 mg (1.5%) at reduced absorption.

Cow's milk contributes between 8% and 4% to calcium balance.

The best foods for calcium balance are those which provide plenty of absorbable calcium while reducing calcium loss. This occurs in fruit and vegetables which provide plenty of potassium which helps retain calcium.

CALCIUM BALANCE

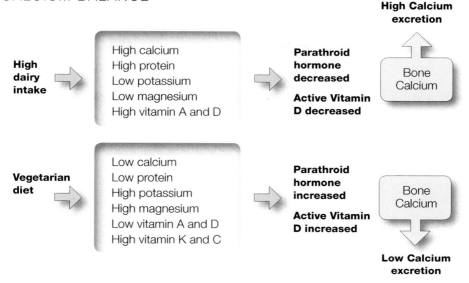

Calcium and Vitamin D

The parathyroid gland is stimulated by a low calcium diet to produce vitamin D in order to aid absorption of calcium.

A high calcium intake suppresses parathyroid activity and vitamin D formation. This means that less of the cholesterol in the skin is converted to vitamin D and may cause a rise in cholesterol levels.

Vitamin D is poorly absorbed from the diet and most is formed by the effect of ultraviolet light or sunshine on the skin.

Vitamin D helps to regulate calcium and phosphate absorption and metabolism which are essential for healthy bones, but it also helps to maintain a healthy immune system by regulating cell growth and differentiation. If less vitamin D is produced there may be an increased risk of cancer

Milk

Cow's milk has a ratio of calcium 10 parts to 1 part of magnesium.

Cheese is over 25 parts calcium to 1 part of magnesium.

The ideal ratio for humans is 2 parts calcium to 1 part of magnesium.

Milk, cheese and other dairy products provide good quality protein and are a good source of calcium. However an excess can cause a relative magnesium deficiency increasing the risk of heart arrhythmias and hypertension.

The high saturated fat content can raise cholesterol levels and increase the risk of cardiovascular disease.

The high protein content can increase the risk of osteoporosis, gout and kidney stones.

Skimmed milk has much less saturated fat but the same amount of calcium and magnesium. Soya milk has almost as much protein but about half the amount of saturated fat and much less calcium (unless added) but an equal amount of magnesium. Nuts, seeds and green leafy vegetables are a good alternative source of calcium and magnesium.

Milk and Children

Cow's milk or cheese is not recommended for children until after six months old. This is because cow's milk differs a great deal from human milk and if given to young children while the gut is immature there is a possibility of the child developing a cow's milk allergy. This produces problems in about one in ten babies. The problems include colic, vomiting, diarrhoea, eczema, asthma, and hyperactivity.

There is also some evidence that type one diabetes is more likely to develop in susceptible babies if given cow's milk in the early months.

Cow's milk is designed for the calf. The average weight of a new born calf is about ten times that of a newborn human child. Cow's milk has a much higher protein, mineral, hormone and saturated fat content than breast milk. The incidence of food allergies is increasing particularly due to wheat and dairy products which make up a large proportion of many teenagers diets.

Avoid an excess of hormones

Sex Hormones and mood swings

Hormonal imbalance may cause mood swings, loss of motivation and depression.

Oestrogen and progesterone deficiency may cause depression. High oestrogen and low progesterone may cause pre-menstrual syndrome with cyclic anxiety and depression.

Testosterone deficiency in both men and women can cause depression, loss of motivation and lack of libido. Testosterone excess may cause hyperactivity and aggression.

These hormones are made from cholesterol and people on very low fat diets often develop hormonal imbalance. We need a reasonable cholesterol intake to make all these hormones. Progesterone is made from cholesterol . A low cholesterol and therefore low progesterone may increase the effect of external oestrogen's.

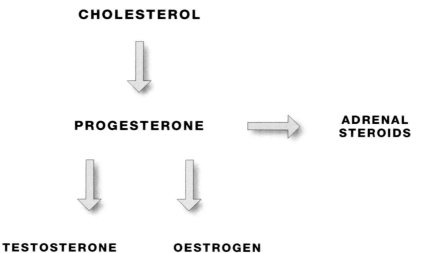

CHOLESTEROL

PROGESTERONE ⟹ **ADRENAL STEROIDS**

TESTOSTERONE **OESTROGEN**

Oestrogen/Progesterone balance

Oestrogen	Progesterone
Stimulates Breast tissue	Maintains breast tissue
Causes cystic breasts	Protects against cystic breast.
Increases risk of breast cancer	Decreases risk of breast cancer.
Stimulates endometrium (lining of the uterus)	Maintains endometrium
Increases risk of endometrial cancer.	Decreases risk of endometrial cancer
Increases risk of Uterine fibroids.	Decreases risk of uterine fibroids.
Slows bone loss	Stimulates bone growth
Increases fluid retention	Decreases fluid retention.
Interferes with thyroid gland	Helps normalise thyroid.
Impairs blood sugar control	Helps blood sugar control.
Increases risk of depression	Decreases risk of depression.
Increases risk of headache	Decreases risk of headache.
Decreases Libido	Increases Libido.
Increases craving and weight gain	Decreases craving and weight gain
Increases fat at hips and thighs	Reduces fat at hips and thighs.

Adapted from "Natural Progesterone" by John Lee. 1996

Oestrogens

A high oestrogen to progesterone ratio increases the risk of fibroids, endometriosis, hypothyroidism, osteoporosis, obesity, depression, fibroadenosis (benign breast lumps), breast, uterine and ovarian cancer.

Sources of environmental/external/strong oestrogen's

The combined contraceptive pill

Hormone Replacement Therapy.

Drinking water containing remnants of the above hormones.

Milk, cheese. yogurt, beef, eggs, fish roe.

Soft plastics:
(Cling film, milk and fruit drink plastic bottles, lining of drink cans)

Some pesticides and detergents.

Some cosmetics e.g. lavender and tea tree oil.

Phytoestrogens.

(Phytoestrogens are weak oestrogen's which are taken up by the body's oestrogen receptors and block the stronger oestrogen's.)

Foods containing phytoestrogens:-

Whole grains, vegetables, soya beans, flax seeds.

Phytoestrogens or natural progesterone may be the most suitable medication for oestrogen deficiency or menopausal symptoms.

Dairy hormones

People in the UK consume on average the equivalent of a pint of milk a day. This includes milk and milk products such as cheese, yogurt and ice cream. Cows also provide meat as in minced beef, steaks, veal and beef burgers.

The life span of a modern cow is about five years rather than the natural 25 to 30 years. During this time they are expected to give birth to a calf every 12 months. After giving birth to a calf they are made pregnant three months later and produce large quantities of milk for nine or ten months of the year. The average milk yield from a cow has increased from 16 pints a day in 1961 to 39 pints in 2004.

During pregnancy the cow's ovaries secrete high levels of progesterone and the placenta secretes high levels of oestrogen. There are also high levels of corticosteroids, growth hormones and prolactin which target the cow's mammary glands to stimulate lactation.

Hormones and chemicals are in much higher concentrations in cow's milk and the meat of cows than in humans.

Recent studies in the UK have shown that about 80% of the dietary intake of female hormones such as oestrogen and progesterone is from dairy produce.

Research has shown that the more oestrogen circulating in the blood the higher the risk of breast cancer.

A group of healthy American women switched from a high fat, low fibre diet (40% of calories as fat and 12g/day of fibre) to a low fat, high fibre diet (20% of calories from fat and 40g/day of fibre).

Within two months their oestrogen levels had dropped by 46%.

Gorbach etc. Nutrition Reviews. Dec. 1992

In the 1980's only 14% of calories in the average Chinese diet were from fat. In America it was 36%. At that time the incidence of breast cancer death was 1 in 10,000 women in rural China and 1 in 10 women in most western countries.

Dairy Oestrogen levels

	Oestradiol-17b
Skimmed milk (non pregnant cow)	5 pg/ml
Whole milk (non pregnant cow)	25 pg/ml
Whole milk (pregnant cow)	85 pg/ml
Fresh and cottage cheese	10 pg/g
Ripened cheese	25 pg/g
Butter	82 pg/g

Cattle Muscle	Heifer (female)	12 pg/g
	Steer (male)	12 pg/g
	Pregnant cow	30 pg/g
Cattle	Liver (Non pregnant female)	40 (male 12) pg/g
	Kidney (Non pregnant female)	40 (male 12) pg/g
	Fat (Non pregnant female)	55 (male 10) pg/g

In cattle given Oestrogen and growth promoting implants to boost growth and milk production, levels of oestradiol were increased by 2 to 4 times.

Other Oestrogen levels

		Oestradiol -17b
Chicken meat (female)		3 to 20 pg/g
Chicken eggs		130 pg/g
Turkey meat (female)		4 pg/g
Fish meat		trace
Fish roe (caviar)		1000 pg/g
Female humans	Serum premenopause	32 – 500 pg/ml
	After oophorectomy (removal of ovaries)	18pg/ml
	Postmenopausal	13pg/ml

Hormone implants including oestrogen, progesterone, testosterone and insulin growth factor have been used in beef and dairy cattle since 1956. They are now used in about 30 countries including the USA, Canada and Australia. Hormone implants have been banned in the European union since 1989. The hormone implants increase the growth rate and amount of muscle compared to fat. They also increase milk yields in dairy cattle. The hormones levels are low in lean muscle but high in meat fat, liver and kidneys. Increased levels are also present in milk, butter and cheese. Often naturally occurring oestrogen levels in milk are high because the cow is pregnant.

Excessive intake of red meat has been associated with an increased risk of breast cancer in humans and this is most likely to be due to oestrogen excess.

Substances produced by cooking meat and growth hormone excess may also be factors.

A high intake of red meat during pregnancy has recently been associated with an increased risk of low sperm counts in the sons of the pregnant mothers.

The Nurses Health Study 2 organised by the Harvard Medical School USA is a study of over 90.000 female nurses aged between 26 years and 46 years starting in 1991. Detailed information about their diets is given by the nurses every four years.

> *Between 1991 and 2003 - 512 women developed breast cancer of the type that is fuelled by oestrogen and progesterone. Women who ate the most red meat had nearly twice the risk of developing these kinds of breast cancer compared with those who ate red meat infrequently.*
>
> **Archives of Internal Medicine . Nov. 2006**

> *"Hormones found in cow's milk include: Oestradiol, Oestriol, Progesterone, Testosterone, 17-Ketosteroids, Corticosterone, Vitamin D, Insulin-like growth factor, growth hormone, prolactin, oxytocin ."*
>
> **Journal of Endocrine Reviews 1992**

The China experience

Until recently the Chinese have had very little milk and dairy products. This is because they have found that the vast majority of Asian people are intolerant to the sugar lactose in milk. Because of their inherited genes they are not able to produce enough of the enzyme lactase that breaks down the sugar in milk from lactose to galactose and glucose.

Their mainly vegetarian diet with no milk and very little meat has meant that they have much less saturated fat, protein and hormones. Their incidence of cardiovascular disease, osteoporosis, mental health problems and cancer is much less than in the west:

	In dairy-free rural china	In the UK
Deaths from breast cancer	1 in 10,000	1 in 10
Deaths from prostate cancer	0.5 in 10,000	1 in 4

In urbanised (westernised) china the deaths from breast cancer increase to 1 in 300.

If people move from China to the West and eat a Western diet the incidence of breast and prostate cancer increases to that in the West showing that the cause of cancer is not usually due to inherited genes but due to environmental and nutritional factors.

Less than 10% of cancers are thought to be made more likely because of your genes and even if a person is at greater risk because of abnormal genes, cancer does not always develop. It will certainly be less likely if you avoid an excess of meat and dairy produce.

High levels of the hormone prolactin are produced by the pregnant cow to increase breast tissue and milk production.

As well as containing high levels of prolactin and oestrogen, cow's milk has high levels of Insulin Growth factor (IGF). It is exactly the same hormone in cows as in humans and stimulates cell division causing an increase in growth and milk production.

IGF (Insulin Growth Factor)

IGF is produced mainly in childhood to stimulate growth.

If IGF levels in the blood increase by 8% the risk of prostate cancer increases seven times.

Levels of IGF in meat and dairy eaters are about 9% higher than in vegans.

*"Serum IGF-1 levels increased significantly in the milk
drinking group... an increase of about 10% above
baseline – but were unchanged in the control group."*

Journal of the American Dietetic Association. 1999

Research in China found that women in the top 25% of IGF scores had two to three times the incidence of breast cancer compared with those in the bottom 25% of IGF scores.

Research from York University UK found that men in the top 25% of IGF levels had three times the risk of prostate cancer.

A number of studies have shown a progressive increase of breast and prostate cancer associated with increasing dairy consumption. Excess oestrogen, IGF and prolactin have all been shown to increase the risk of breast and prostate cancer.

The growth and spread of cancer is often reduced by hormonal treatment. Anti-oestrogen drugs such as tamoxifen, anastrozole and letrozole may also reduce IGF. Progesterones such as megestrol acetate are also helpful in reducing the relative excess of oestrogen.

In men, anti-androgen treatment reduces the growth and spread of prostate cancer. Gonadorelin analogue injections such as Zoladex and Prostap may reduce both IGF and androgen levels.

As well as these anti-hormone treatments it would seem sensible to advise patients to reduce the intake of dietary hormones by reducing their intake of meat and milk products from cows.

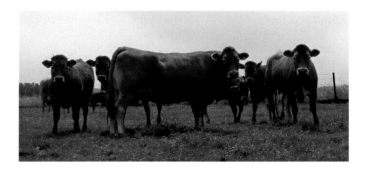

Dairy

Milk which comes from an animal that is much larger than ourselves and usually pregnant -contains high levels of the following:

Content		Associated with
Hormones	Oestrogen	Breast, ovarian and colon cancer, fibroids, endometriosis, hypothyroidism.
	Androgens	Acne, prostate cancer
	Corticosteroids	Endometrial and breast cancer, osteoporosis.
	Insulin Growth factor	Diabetes, acne, breast and prostate cancer.
	Leptin	Obesity.
	Thyroxine	Possible thyroid problems
	Prolactin	Breast and prostate cancer
Saturated fatty acids		Cardiovascular disease, Gallstones
Protein		Osteoporosis, Renal stones, high homocysteine, eczema, asthma, allergies, indigestion and peptic ulcers
Lactose/Galactose		Irritable bowel, cataracts, glaucoma.
High Calcium/Low Magnesium		Hypertension, heart arrhythmias.

Cow's meat and milk products
Should they carry a health warning?

I have very carefully considered the evidence for and against cow's meat and milk products. The dairy industry has been extremely successful and expert in promoting its products. I have great admiration for dairy farmers who I am sure are well intentioned, hard working and inadequately rewarded for a very responsible and difficult job. I am sure that as with the general public they have been sold the message that dairy products are good for if not vital for our health.

Cigarette smoking was suspected to be responsible for an increased risk of cardiovascular disease and cancer for many years before an independent scientist was able to persuade the government that the risk was genuine. Despite strong evidence the powerful cigarette industry denied any problem and increased its marketing efforts in the third world countries to maintain its profits.

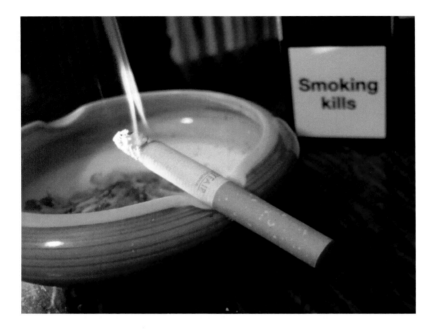

As with smoking it is very difficult to provide definite evidence that cow's meat or milk is responsible for poor health as it is only one of many other factors. However I am increasingly convinced that, after smoking tobacco, consuming an excess of cow's meat, milk, cheese and milk products is the next greatest hazard to good health.

Following recent books suggesting this possibility, I suspect the dairy industry is already aware of the possible decrease in sales in western countries and has tried to maintain its profits by increasing its efforts in poorer and less informed countries.

Eat grass fed (organic) meat, dairy products and eggs.

Meat from grass fed cattle has, compared to grain fed:

- About one third less saturated fat.
- About four times more Omega-3 and CLA fatty acids
- About four times more vitamin E and beta-carotene (vitamin A)
- A lot more magnesium, which is in chlorophyll.

Omega-3 fatty acids are most abundant in seafood and certain nuts and seeds such as walnuts and flaxseeds, but they are also found in animals who feed on grass. Omega-3 is formed in the chloroplasts of green leaves and algae.

Over half of the fatty acids in grass are Omega-3 .

Less than one quarter of the fatty acids in grain is omega-3.

Meat, milk, butter, cheese and eggs all contain much more omega-3, CLA and vitamin E if the cows, pig, sheep, turkey or chicken are fed on grass. Eggs from grass fed chickens contain as much as ten times more omega-3 than factory hens kept indoors and fed on grain.

CLA (conjugated linoleic acid) is like omega-3 - a 'good fat'. Grass fed animals contain about four times more CLA than grain fed. Hay feeding is not as effective because some of the fatty acids are oxidised in the drying of the grass.

CLA seems to help prevent cancer, atheroma and immune disorders. A study in Finland showed that women with the highest levels of CLA had a 60% lower risk of breast cancer than those with the lowest levels.

Meat from grass fed cattle is about four times higher in vitamin E than grain fed. Vitamin E reduces the risk of cardiovascular disease and cancer. It also increases fertility and reduces aging.

Cud-chewing ruminant animals such as cows and sheep are designed to live outside in the sunshine and eat fibrous grasses, plants, herbs and shrubs and not live indoors eating low fibre starchy grain such as corn, soya beans and various other foods such as restaurant waste. The animals fed abnormal diets are prone to illness and often require antibiotics.

In the UK, because of the weather, most dairy cattle are only grass fed and receiving sunshine for less than six months of the year. The resulting meat and milk has less important nutrients such as Omega-3, vitamin D, magnesium and phytonutrients unless these are provided in the feed.

I believe there has been more attention paid to animal feeding since the 'mad cow' disease scare and there have been improvements such as avoiding animal products and adding more omega-3 oils such as rapeseed to the feed.

One of the reasons the Mediterranean diet produces less illness of all kinds is probably because, as well as eating less meat and dairy products than their more northern European neighbours, their animals, which are usually sheep, goats and chicken rather than cows, spend much more time in the sunshine eating grass and a greater variety of plants and herbs.

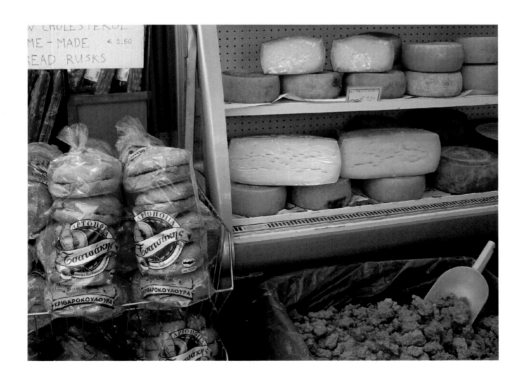

Avoid too much saturated fat and a high cholesterol diet.

Saturated fat

All animal and vegetable fats are a mixture of saturated and unsaturated fats but the proportions vary. Animals store fat as mainly saturated fat and therefore eating a lot of meat or dairy products gives a high intake of saturated fat.

Excess sugar and protein ingested is converted into saturated fat and stored in the body.

A certain amount of saturated fat is necessary to help the essential fatty acids to be more effective.

It also contains important fat soluble vitamins (A, D, E and K.)

An excess of saturated fat easily causes obesity as fat contains twice as many calories as carbohydrate or protein.

An excess of saturated fat and cholesterol increases the risk of gallstones as excess cholesterol is excreted through the gallbladder.

An excess of saturated fat and red meat is associated with an increased risk of cancer.

An excess of saturated fat increases the blood cholesterol especially LDL "the bad cholesterol". It therefore increases the risk of atherosclerosis and cardiovascular disease.

Atherosclerosis

Atherosclerosis causes furring up or blocking of arteries and is the major cause of illness and death in western countries. It was very rare until about eighty years ago. It is not seen in wild animals and is rare in third world countries that have a more primitive diet.

- In the brain or neck (carotids) it causes strokes and dementia.
- In the heart (coronary) arteries it causes heart attacks and heart failure.

- In the aortic artery it causes aneurysms
- In the Intestinal arteries it causes constipation and bowel problems.
- In the arteries to the kidneys it causes hypertension and renal failure.
- In the pelvic and leg arteries it causes leg pain and poor circulation.

Our knowledge of the process that takes place in atherosclerosis is complicated and incomplete.

The process seems to start with fissure type damage to the arterial wall where there is maximum turbulence and stress. Damage is more likely to occur if the artery is unhealthy. This may occur when there is a lack of antioxidants or an excess of oxidants. Oxidants include cigarette smoke, trans-fats, raised homocysteine and various toxins. Antioxidants such as Vitamin C and E , selenium, zinc, carotenoids, lycopene and Omega-3 are known to be important but other nutrients are probably also involved.

As a reaction to the injury to the arterial wall a thrombus forms over the fissure or wound. This includes platelets, fibrin, lipoproteins containing cholesterol, red and white blood cells. To prevent the clot breaking free like a wound scab it is rapidly covered by a thin layer of endothelial cells and incorporated into the artery wall. Further injury and repeated thrombosis may occur causing increasing narrowing of the artery. A lack of essential nutrients may delay the healing and make the plaque liable to rupture causing a massive thrombotic episode which blocks the artery and results in a heart attack, stroke or blocked artery elsewhere.

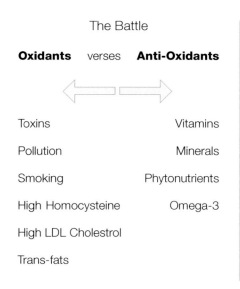

The Battle

Oxidants   verses   **Anti-Oxidants**

Oxidants	Anti-Oxidants
Toxins	Vitamins
Pollution	Minerals
Smoking	Phytonutrients
High Homocysteine	Omega-3
High LDL Cholestrol	
Trans-fats	

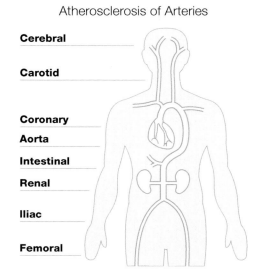

Atherosclerosis of Arteries

Cerebral

Carotid

Coronary

Aorta

Intestinal

Renal

Iliac

Femoral

Pauling's theory

Dr Linus Pauling was one of the most important scientists of his day and the only man to win two individual Nobel prizes (For Chemistry in 1954 and Peace in 1962). He wrote 'A Unified Theory of Human Cardiovascular Disease' in 1992 when over 90 years of age.

He noted that, unlike man, most animals make vitamin C in their bodies. For example an adult goat weighing 60Kg produces 13,000mg of vitamin C a day. About 40 million years ago man's ancestors are thought to have lost the ability to synthesise vitamin C from glucose in their bodies because they could get enough from their food. At that time there was a plentiful supply of fruit and plant material to compensate.

When our ancestors left tropical regions and in ice ages, vegetation was scarce and there was a high risk of scurvy. To prevent leaking arteries from vitamin C deficiency we may have developed the ability to deposit lipoprotein A along artery walls at times of vitamin C deficiency.

Lipoprotein A can repair damaged or leaky arteries but it increases the risk of heart disease by building up deposits on artery walls.

Linus Pauling believed this was one of the causes of atherosclerosis and advised a large intake of vitamin C. He advised huge doses of 18,000 mg daily but research by the Linus Pauling Institute has suggested that no more than 200 mg is absorbable in one day. The present recommended daily allowance is 60 to 100 mg daily.

Vitamin C is a powerful antioxidant which reduces LDL and raises HDL cholesterol. It reduces Lipoprotein A levels in the blood. It decreases blood stickiness which reduces the risk of thrombosis and hypertension.

Causes of Atherosclerosis

- The rise in saturated fat consumption mainly from red meat and dairy products.
- The increase in LDL cholesterol levels and decrease in HDL cholesterol levels.
- The increase in processed and deep fried food containing Trans-fats.
- The lack of omega-3 fatty acids.
- The excess of omega-6 over omega-3.(20 to 1; Ideal 2 to 1)

- The excess of animal protein causing raised homocysteine levels.
- The huge rise in sugar consumption with very little essential nutrients.
- The increase in obesity.
- The reduction in exercise because of new technology such as motor transport, washing machines etc.
- The introduction of refined wheat grain with removal of nutritious wheat germ. (vitamin E, chromium, magnesium, essential fatty acids and fibre)
- The increase of cooking, reducing infection but also reducing many nutrients.
- Vitamin C deficiency due to a reduction in raw fresh fruit and vegetables.
- The increase in exposure to oxidants such as carbon monoxide and pollutants due to rise in cigarette smoking and motor transport.
- The introduction of chlorination of water supplies to stop water borne infection and the use of chlorine dioxide to bleach and disinfect white flour.
- The increase in exposure to other oxidants such as industrial waste, pesticides, weed killers, detergents, cosmetics etc.

Cholesterol

Cholesterol is a type of fat found in all of us. It is an essential compound necessary for the making of body cells and hormones. Our body makes its own cholesterol in the liver and only about 30% is supplied by food.

Cholesterol is only found in animal foods. Some people are sensitive to cholesterol in foods while others have a minimal response to dietary intake.

Cholesterol is transported around the body by lipoproteins.

"Bad" LDL (Low Density Lipoprotein) is the most common lipoprotein and although some is essential, too much can fur up the arteries.

"Good" HDL (High Density Lipoprotein) makes up about a third of the lipoproteins in our blood. It carries excess cholesterol away from our arteries and back to the liver.

A genetic condition which causes high cholesterol (familial hypercholesterolemia) occurs in about 1 in 500 people in the UK.

The risk of coronary heart disease increases as the person's cholesterol increases.

- The average UK cholesterol level in 1993 was about 6 mmol/L.
- The average level has fallen since this time due to dietary advice and the greater use of statins.
- Ideally your total cholesterol should be about 5 mmol/l.
- LDL (bad) cholesterol should be below 3 mmol/l
- HDL (good) cholesterol should be above 1.5 mmol/l
- The best predictor of risk for heart disease is the total cholesterol/HDL ratio. This should be below 4 indicating that over a quarter of your cholesterol is of HDL (good) cholesterol.

Elevated triglyceride levels also increase the risk of atherosclerosis.

Fats and Cholesterol

Bad Fats

Saturated fats- raise LDL and triglycerides and lower HDL (In dairy products, red meat, coconut oil, palm oil).

Trans-fats - raise LDL and triglycerides and lower HDL (partially hydrogenated vegetable oil in margarine, biscuits, cakes, pastries, pies, sausages, ready meals. etc.)

Good Fats

Polyunsaturated fats – Lower LDL and triglycerides and have no effect or increase HDL .

Omega 3- Oily fish, walnuts, seeds of flax (linseed) mustard and pumpkin, leafy green plants and vegetables.

Omega-6 - sunflower, safflower and corn oil, sesame seeds.

Monounsaturated fats – Lower LDL and triglycerides and have no effect on or increase HDL

Omega-9 - Olive oil, Rapeseed, Avocado, nuts.

All animal and plant products have a mixture of fats.

	Total fat per 100g	Saturated Fat	Mono unsaturated	Poly unsaturated
Olive oil	100g	14g	70g	11g
Butter	82g	54g	21g	3g
Margarine	82g	16g	21g	41g (6.0g trans)
Bertolli	59g	14g	30g	14g (0.5g trans)
Flora Pro-active	35g	8g	9g	17g (0.5g trans)
Cheddar cheese	34g	22g	10g	1g
Avocado	20g	4g	12g	2g
Eggs	11g	3g	5g	1g
Whole milk	3g	2g	1g	0g

Cholesterol

Cholesterol is essential for health.

- It protects the structure of cell membranes.
- It is important for nerve conduction.
- It is essential for the production of sex and adrenal hormones.
- It is essential for the production of vitamin D from the skin.
- It is essential for the production of bile acids in the gallbladder which then help in the absorption of fat and fat soluble vitamins.(A,D,E and K).

Very low cholesterol levels (below 4mmol/l) are associated with less coronary heart disease but an increased overall mortality. Very low cholesterols have been associated with poor memory, depression, strokes, and cancer.

Lowering cholesterol by diet – Plant Sterols

A diet high in fruits, vegetables and wholegrain foods provides plant sterols and stanols (plant fats or phytosterols) which lower cholesterol.

Plant sterols and stanols have a similar molecular structure to cholesterol but they inhibit intestinal absorption of animal fat Cholesterol.

The American Journal of Medicine reviewed 16 published trials that gave plant sterols and stanols to almost 600 people.

- Total cholesterol was lowered by 10%.
- LDL (bad cholesterol) lowered by 13%

People who in addition ate plant-sterol-enriched margarines:

- Total cholesterol lowered by 18%.
- LDL lowered by 23%

How to reduce LDL Cholesterol

Reduce intake of saturated and trans fats. e.g. dairy products and red meat, hard margarine, biscuits, cakes.

Reduce intake of protein. Excess is converted to sugar and fat.

Reduce intake of sugar. Excess causes fat and raised LDL.

Increase cholesterol-lowering foods:

Polyunsaturated fats – Omega-3 in Oily fish, walnuts, flaxseeds, green leafy plants. Omega-6 in plant and seed oils

Monounsaturated fats- avocados, olive oil, nuts.

Plant sterols and fibre - fruit, vegetables, wholegrain foods

Foods rich in soluble fibre- oats, barley, beans, peas, apples.

Soya beans

Garlic

Nicotinic acid (Niacin) – vitamin B in cereal, bread, nuts..

Total cholesterol can be reduced by medication:

Simvastatin 10 mg reduces LDL by about 30%,

Simvastatin 40 mg reduces LDL by about 40%,

Nicotinic acid (Niacin or Vit.B3) reduces LDL by about 25% (in meat, white bread and cereals which are fortified)

However LDL cholesterol can also be reduced by weight loss (especially if this involves a reduction in saturated fat from animal meat and dairy products) and by a careful choice of foods.

Weight loss of 8Kg or 10% reduces LDL by about 20%.

Plant sterols reduce it by about 10 to 20%

A bowl of oatmeal reduces it by about 10 to 20%

Soya foods reduce it by about 10%

Nuts reduce cholesterol by about 10% but reduce cardiovascular risk by about 30% probably because they contain essential fatty acids and magnesium.

How to raise HDL

HDL is raised by:

Monounsaturated fatty acids- olive oil, avocado and nuts.

Omega-3 fatty acids – oily fish, green plants.

Vitamin B3 (niacin or nicotinic acid)- nuts, meat, bread.

Vitamin C (fruit and vegetables)

Alcohol

Exercise

Stopping smoking

Drugs that raise HDL :

Niacin increases HDL by 30%.

Statins increase HDL by 5 to 20%.

Ezetimibe increases HDL by only 3%.

Combination of Statin and Niacin may give best lipid profile.

How to reduce triglycerides

Reduce total fat intake especially saturated animal fats – butter, cream, cheese, fatty meats, pastries, biscuits and cakes made with butter.

Increase relative proportion of Omega-3 fatty acids such as in oily fish which reduce triglycerides.

Reduce sugar and other high–GI foods which raise triglycerides. Avoid sugar and sweet foods such as biscuits, cakes, chocolate, Cola-like drinks and ice creams. Eat low-GI foods- fruit, vegetables, bread and pasta.

Have small frequent meals rather than one or two large ones.

Reduce alcohol which raises triglycerides.

Gallstones

A high saturated fat intake and related high cholesterol are a major cause of gallstones. In the western world, by the age of 60 years, almost 30% of men and women have gallstones. Each year more than 500,000 Americans have gallbladder surgery.

In Asia and Africa gallstones are rare. Denis Burkitt noted that "In 20 years of surgery in Africa, I had to remove exactly one gallstone."

A more vegetarian diet with high fibre and low fat content are the most likely factors in the reduced incidence.

The loss of your gallbladder reduces your ability to produce sufficient bile acids to digest and absorb fats and fat soluble vitamins. It also reduces the excretion of cholesterol and may cause a rise in blood cholesterol levels.

Avoid Trans-fats

In the 1860s a cattle plague caused butter prices to rise and a cheaper butter substitute was looked for. One of the first was made from blubber and milk. After 1900 margarine was developed. It was made by bubbling hydrogen through polyunsaturated vegetable oil which made it solidify. The product was easily spread, cheap and had a long shelf life.

In the 1950s margarine became more popular than butter as nutritionists and doctors advised that vegetable oils with polyunsaturated fat were better for your health than butter with saturated fat. Unfortunately it was not realised that the processing of vegetable fats changed some of them from a cis-form which helps to build membranes and hormones into a trans-form which tends to block the good fatty acids and have a harmful effect on cells and prostaglandin hormones.

Some trans-fats occur naturally in meat and dairy products. They are also formed when vegetable oils are exposed to excess heat and light during extraction. Omega-3 polyunsaturated fats are the most unstable and easily convert to trans-fats. Omega-6 is slightly more stable. Monounsaturated and saturated fats are the most stable and least likely to form trans-fats. There is therefore an advantage in using saturated fat such as palm oil or cold-pressed monounsaturated fat such as olive oil in cooking and using cold-pressed polyunsaturated fats such as flax seed oil or monounsaturated fats such as olive oil as salad dressing or on bread as a substitute for butter or margarine.

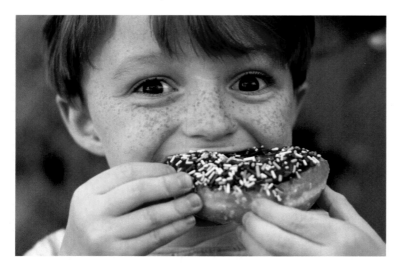

Today most vegetable oils are extracted from hard seeds with heat, pressure and chemical solvents which create trans-fatty acids. Trans- fatty acids are created in abundance by the process of partial hydrogenation in which the vegetable oil is heated to high temperatures with hydrogen gas under pressure for several hours. When you deep-fry foods the oil reaches high temperatures and some of the oil is oxidised or converted into trans-fats. If re-used the oil becomes increasingly oxidised (rancid) and the concentration of trans-fats gradually increases.

Trans-fats are now known to be powerful oxidants which, unless opposed by sufficient anti-oxidants, can damage arterial and body cells and DNA. This increases the risk of atherosclerosis, cardiovascular disease and inflammatory disease including arthritis and cancer.

Trans-fats block the conversion of essential fats into vital brain fats such as DHA, GLA and prostaglandins. This causes an increased risk of poor memory and concentration, attention deficit disorder, dementia, depression and other mental disorders.

Trans-fats increase LDL (the bad cholesterol) and reduce HDL (the good cholesterol).

Studies showed people who ate margarine with high levels of trans-fats were at higher risk of developing heart disease than those who ate butter. Above average consumption of trans-fats doubles the risk of a heart attack.

A study of 120,000 NHS nurses reviewed by the New England Journal of Medicine in 2006 found that the risk of heart disease doubled for every 19% rise in natural fat intake while the same risk doubled for every 2% rise in trans-fat intake.

The incidence of heart attacks, stroke and cancer rose dramatically in the 1950s and 1960s. It is suspected that the introduction of partially hydrogenated vegetable oils and trans-fats in margarine, biscuits, cakes and pastry, as well as the popularity of crisps and deep fried chips was a major contributing factor. The increase in smoking at this time was another factor.

Trans-fats are present in margarine, crisps, biscuits, cakes, chocolate and cereal bars, doughnuts, pies, pastries, pizza, chocolates, ice cream and ready meals. They are created in any food which is deep fried.

They are listed in ingredients as hydrogenated vegetable fat or partly hydrogenated fat or oil.

Trans fats have no nutritional benefits and disrupt the absorption of beneficial essential fatty acids.

The World Health Organisation's recommended intake is zero.

- We consume an average of 3g trans fats per day.
- A bag of crisps gives you 4g of trans fats.
- A serving of French fries or fried fish gives you 8g.
- A doughnut gives you 12g.

It is estimated that the average total fat intake of an American man is 150 to 250g a day and trans-fats may be up to 25% of this.

- Recommended intake of total fat is 70 to 100g.
- Recommended intake of trans-fats is nil.

Unfortunately trans-fats are about 80% cheaper than natural saturated fats such as butter and palm oil and so are widely used as a substitute.

Fat improves the taste of food and preserves it so that the item has a very long shelf life. Over the last few years there has been increasing pressure on food manufacturers to declare the amount of trans-fats present in items of food and there is a welcome and increasing threat of legislation to limit the use of trans-fats.

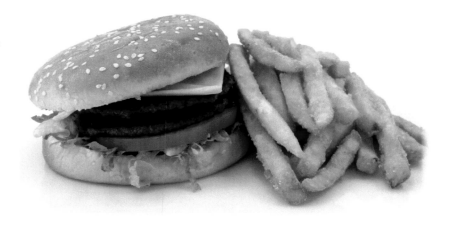

Have adequate essential fatty acids
with correct ratio of omega-3 to omega-6

Essential fatty acids are present in green plants, fruit, wheat germ, seeds, nuts and fish. Plants can synthesize omega-3 and omega-6 fatty acids from glucose but animals can only synthesize saturated fatty acids from glucose. Animals need to eat these essential fatty acids for normal metabolism and can store them.

Most seeds such as corn and beans such as soya contain mainly Omega-6 as it is more stable to store. The chloroplasts in green algae (plankton) in the sea, and green leafy plants on land, can convert Omega-6 to Omega-3 so that they have the correct ratio of fatty acids.

Fish cannot make omega-3 but if they feed on plant algae in the sea they will have stores of omega-3. The omega-3 content of farmed fish is very dependant on what they get to eat. Often the feed contains mainly omega-6 grain.

Animals that graze on grass or green vegetables will have stores of omega-3 and omega-6 fatty acids in the correct ratio. However if they are animals or birds such as chickens confined to barns and fed corn or other cereals their meat and eggs will contain mainly omega-6 and very little omega-3.

All plants have a mixture of omega-3 and omega-6 but the relative amounts vary:

	Polyunsaturated fat		Saturated and Monounsaturated fat
	Omega-6	Omega-3	
Flaxseed	15%	50%	35%
Hempseed	55%	20%	25%
Walnuts	55%	15%	30%
Rapeseed oil	20%	10%	70%
Wheat germ	55%	7%	38%
Olive oil	9%	1%	90%
Corn oil	58%	1%	41%
Sunflower seed	65%	0%	35%

Essential Fats

Polyunsaturated fats such as omega-3 and 6 are essential because the body cannot manufacture them and so they must be obtained from the diet. Omega-6 is abundant in the western diet but most people are deficient in omega-3.

The ideal balance is thought to be about 2 to 4 times more omega-6 than omega-3. The present western diet contains 15 to 25 times more omega-6 than omega-3.

Too much omega-6 promotes an inflammatory state increasing the risk of cardiovascular disease and many other disorders.

A deficiency of omega-3 means the body cannot build an ideal cell membrane. This increases the risk of cardiovascular disease, insulin resistance, diabetes, asthma, hypertension, macular degeneration, auto-immune disorders, osteoarthritis, attention deficit/hyperactivity, depression and some cancers. Deficiency causes vague symptoms such as dry skin, fatigue, constipation, brittle nails and hair, frequent infections, poor concentration, depression and joint pains.

There has been a major shift over the last 100 years in the ratio of omega-6 to omega-3 fatty acids. The dietary intake has changed from a ratio of 1 to 1 on the African plains to between 10 to 1 and 25 to 1 in the US today. According to research by the charities Mental Health Foundation and Sustain in their report 'Feeding Minds' 2006 this imbalance has resulted in increases in depression, as well as concentration and memory problems.

The report notes that there has been a 34% decline in vegetable consumption and a 59% drop in the amount of fish eaten over the last 60 years. Only 13% of men and 15% of women now eat at least five portions of fruit and vegetables a day.

Prostaglandins

History

Professor Ulf von Euler from Sweden in 1935 showed that seminal fluid in man and animals contained a substance that influenced blood vessels and muscle fibres. He called the substance prostaglandin. He won the Nobel Prize for Physiology and Medicine in 1970 for his fundamental discoveries in the role of hormones and neurotransmitters.

In 1982 the Nobel Prize for Physiology and Medicine was won by Sune Bergstrom and Bengt Samuelsson from Sweden and John Vane from England. They had purified the first prostaglandins and determined their structure and actions. They also established that unsaturated, essential fatty acids formed the parent substances for this system and that aspirin worked by inhibiting prostaglandins.

The prostaglandins formed part of a newly discovered biological system which regulated a number of vital life processes. They were described as defence hormones as they were constantly being formed in the blood vessel walls and blood cells to counter infection, allergies, inflammation and thrombosis.

Omega-6 and omega-3 are essential to form prostaglandins.

Prostaglandins are hormone like substances which control the movement of calcium and other substances in and out of cells. This enables them to regulate most physiological functions such as:

- Inflammatory response.
- Immune response.
- Blood coagulation.
- Pain.
- Fever.
- Sleep.
- Smooth muscle contraction of bowel, uterus etc.
- Contraction and relaxation of arteries.
- Contraction and relaxation of bronchi.
- Stomach acid production.
- Cell growth and division.
- Sexual function.

Imbalance of prostaglandins may be a major factor in:

- Osteoarthritis.
- Asthma and allergies.
- Hypertension.
- Thrombosis including heart attacks and strokes.
- Peptic ulcers and Inflammatory bowel disease.
- Inflammatory bowel disease
- Depression, chronic fatigue and mental health disorders.
- Attention deficit, poor memory and dementia
- Skin problems such as eczema and psoriasis.
- Glaucoma, macular degeneration and eye problems.
- Diabetes.
- Neurological disorders.
- Miscarriage and infertility.
- Autoimmune disease
- Cancer.

OMEGA 6		OMEGA 3
Linoleic acid (Corn, maize, safflower, sunflower, sesame and margarines based on these oils. Most seeds and nuts, peanuts, Soy beans, meat if fed on corn and other grains.)		**alpha - linolenic acid** (Plankton, oils of flax (linseed), walnuts, berries, rapeseed oil, pumpkin seeds, hempseed. Dark leafy greens and grasses, purslane. Oily fish such as mackerel, sardines, salmon. Meat if fed on grass and plants.)
GLA (Evening primrose, blackcurrant)		
DGLA (Liver and animal organs)	**Arachidonic acid (AA)** (Meat, milk, butter, eggs if chicken fed on grain.)	**EPA and DHA** (Fish, fish oils, liver, human milk, eggs if chicken fed on grass.)
Prostaglandin 1 (Anti-inflammatory)	**Prostaglandin 2** (Inflammatory)	**Prostaglandin 3** (Anti-inflammatory)

Enzymes for both pathways require:
Vitamins B6, B3, B12, biotin, C, E and zinc.

Prostaglandin 1 and 3 are anti-inflammatory. They :

Reduce blood coagulation,
Dilate blood vessels and reduce blood pressure,
Decrease inflammation and pain,
Maintain water electrolyte balance,
Dilate bronchi,
Inhibit gastric secretion,
Improve nerve and immune function.
Help insulin work.

Prostaglandins 1 and 3 are essential for proper brain function affecting vision, learning ability, coordination and mood.

Arachidonic acid is essential for brain function but excess can promote inflammation rather than reduce it. It produces Prostaglandin 2 which is inflammatory and can produce the reverse effects of Prostaglandin 1 and 3. The inflammatory effect including pain is opposed by non steroidal anti-inflammatory drugs (NSAIDS) such as ibuprofen.

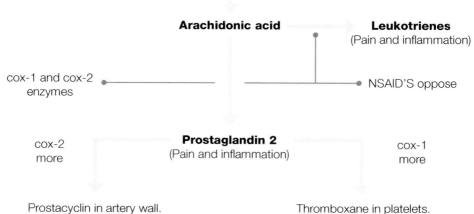

OMEGA-6, MEAT AND DAIRY PRODUCTS

Arachidonic acid → **Leukotrienes**
(Pain and inflammation)

cox-1 and cox-2 enzymes

NSAID'S oppose

cox-2
more

Prostaglandin 2
(Pain and inflammation)

cox-1
more

Prostacyclin in artery wall.
Causes dilatation of artery, inhibits platelet clumping, anti- thrombosis.

Thromboxane in platelets.
Causes constriction of artery, platelet clumping, pro-thrombosis, protects stomach lining (prostacyclin in gut), protects kidney function.

However, as can be seen from the diagram, inflammation could also be reduced by having more omega-3, less omega-6 and less arachidonic acid producers such as meat and dairy products. Trans-fats have the effect of reducing the anti-inflammatory prostaglandins and increasing the effect of the inflammatory prostaglandin.

Although prostaglandin 2 can be inflammatory it tries to keep a balance between the thromboxane and prostacyclin that it produces.

Pregnancy and childhood

Several studies show that women who consume diets rich in omega-3 fatty acids have longer gestations and babies of higher birth weight than those on diets low in these fatty acids.

During pregnancy a woman's brain is used as a source of fatty acids to help build the baby's brain. The mother's brain may shrink by 3% unless she has a sufficient intake of omega-3 fatty acids.. If she then breastfeeds she will continue to lose fatty acids on a daily basis.

An analysis of more than 14,000 women from over 20 countries showed that a higher intake of omega-3 fatty acids from seafood was associated with a lower incidence of postnatal depression.

Children born to mothers who had a high omega-3 fatty acid intake **scored** higher in intelligence tests at the age of 4 years.

Infants weaned from breast milk to a formula milk that was supplemented with omega-3 fatty acids had significantly better visual acuity at 17, 26 and 52 weeks of age than infants weaned to a milk supplemented without omega-3 fatty acids.

Adequate intake of omega 3 reduces the risk of eczema and asthma.

Essential fats are very important in brain development. One quarter of brain weight is DHA.(Docosahexaenoic acid) derived from omega-3 (linolenic acid). 30% of the dry weight of the retina is made up of fatty acids, mainly DHA. These same fatty acids are also the major constituents of the membranes that surround every single cell in the human body. DHA is especially important in pregnancy and infancy as it is used to build and develop the brain.

DHA is present in breast milk and the World Health Organisation now recommends that formula feeds include these essential oils.

Research at Hammersmith hospital in London, UK suggests that a high intake of polyunsaturated fat rather than saturated fat increases intelligence. Babies of vegan breast feeding mothers were brighter on average than formula fed babies or babies breast fed by mothers with a high saturated fat intake and low intake of essential fatty acids.

The Eskimo diet

Dr Hugh Macdonald Sinclair FRCP while serving in the British army during World War Two and involved in nutritional research, observed that there was a very low incidence of heart disease among Eskimo populations. This was surprising as their diet was extremely high in fat and extremely low in fruit and vegetables. He concluded that the type of fat in their diet must help to keep them healthy.

Using himself as a guinea pig, Sinclair ate only seal and fish for 100 days. He demonstrated a remarkable decrease in his clotting time when he cut his skin. In 1956 in a letter published in the Lancet, he claimed that most of the world's so called "Diseases of civilization" – coronary heart disease, cancer, diabetes, inflammation, strokes and skin disease- were caused by a disturbance in fat metabolism. This was not well received by the medical profession at that time but subsequent research has vindicated his theories.

Sinclair theorized that the major reason for the disturbance in fat metabolism was because the typical Western diet was full of processed foods, saturated fats and trans-fatty acids ("bad fats") which blocked the "good fats". He called these good fats essential fatty acids (EFAs) because the body cannot make them for itself and must obtain them from food.

Today we know that essential fatty acids are vital to the construction of every cell of the body, including the brain. Like vitamins and minerals they are essential for the proper function of enzymes, hormones and prostaglandins.

Current research demonstrates low levels of essential fats in many cases of attention deficit disorder, Parkinson's disease, Alzheimer's disease, depression, behavioural disorders such as aggression, autism, autoimmune disease, asthma, eczema, multiple sclerosis, alcoholism and cancer.

Omega 3 and cardiovascular disease

Effects of omega-3:

Improves health and elasticity of arteries.
Lowers blood pressure.
Lowers triglycerides.
Raises HDL the "good" cholesterol. (anti-atherogenic)
Reduces the risk of arrhythmias. (anti-arrhythmic)
Reduces the stickiness of platelets. (anti-thrombotic)

Because of these effects it reduces the risk of Hypertension and Cardiovascular disease

Advice on diet to produce correct balance of prostaglandins.

- Avoid hydrogenated fats (trans-fats).
- Avoid excess of processed omega-6 vegetable oils, (e.g. soy, corn, cottonseed and sesame seeds).
- Have wholegrain bread which unlike white bread has essential fatty acids and also essential vitamins and minerals.
- Have green vegetables and have meat and eggs from grass fed animals and poultry for omega 3
- Eat pulses (beans and peas)
- Eat some nuts including walnuts and seeds.
- Avoid refined sugar and corn syrup.
- Eat occasional organic poultry eggs and muscle meat.
- Eat fish or shellfish.
- Eat organ meats and fish eggs occasionally.
- Use small amounts of good quality butter, olive oil or low trans fat spreads instead of margarine.
- Use olive oil, rapeseed oil or coconut oil in cooking.
- Use flax oil in salad dressings.

Have sufficient, but avoid an excess of, fat-soluble vitamins.

The fat soluble vitamins are stored in fat and if taken in excess can cause toxic effects. This compares with water soluble vitamins which even in excess rarely cause any toxic effects.

The fat soluble vitamins are:

Vitamin A
Vitamin D
Vitamin E
Vitamin K

Vitamin A

Vitamin A is essential for the health of the eye and the immune system. It has an important role in bone growth, reproduction, cell division and cell differentiation. It helps maintain and protect from infection the surface linings of the eyes, lungs, urinary tract, intestinal tract, mucous membranes and skin.

Vitamin A deficiency contributes to blindness by making the cornea very dry and easily damaged. It also causes damage to the retina. Night blindness is an early sign of deficiency. In developing countries at least three million children a year develop xeropthalmia due to vitamin A deficiency. Damage to the cornea of the eye and retina causes about half a million children to go blind. Also millions of children die from the complications of infectious diseases such as measles, enteritis and chest infections. Their resistance to infection is reduced by vitamin A deficiency. Vitamin A deficiency decreases bone development and bone growth leading to short stature.

Excess of vitamin A may cause:

Birth defects
Liver abnormalities
Reduced bone density and osteoporosis

Most cases result from excess of vitamin A supplements or excess cod liver oil but may occur if very large amounts of liver, fatty meat, dairy products or carrots are consumed. Acute toxicity causes nausea, vomiting, headache, dizziness, blurred vision and poor muscular coordination.

Research in Sweden showed that women with twice recommended intake of vitamin A had reduced bone density and increased risk of hip fracture as compared with women who consumed less than recommended intake. (Study of 72,000 postmenopausal women.)

Another study of 2000 Swedish men showed that the risk of fracture was greatest in men with high retinol (vitamin A) levels. The risk was seven times greater in men with the highest levels.

Vitamin A is fat soluble and stored in the body fat where it may accumulate until required. Recommended daily intake is 600 mcg for women and 700 mcg for men.

An intake greater than 1500 mcg is associated with Osteoporosis.

There are two types of Vitamin A.

- Retinol - preformed in animal foods such as milk, cheese, eggs, fish and Liver. Fish liver oils are the richest source of retinol.
- Carotenes - in red, yellow and green fruits and vegetables such as spinach, carrots, peppers, peaches and apricots.

Carotenes are converted to retinol by the body but it takes 6 grams of carotene to make one gram of retinol.

A diet containing five portions of fruit and vegetables a day and including dark green leafy vegetables, yellow or orange fruits provides adequate vitamin A.

On a vegetarian diet it is difficult to exceed the recommended intake of vitamin A but on a diet rich in animal products it is very easy, especially as there may be a high amount of stored vitamin A from previous meals.

The recommended daily intake is 800mcg.

An average portion of...	supplies (mcg)
Calf's liver	10,000
Liver pate	5,800
Two egg omelette	1,200
Boiled egg	70
Cheddar cheese	140
Double cream (tablespoon)	200
Full fat Cows milk (half pint)	160
Skimmed milk (half pint)	3
Shepherd's pie	450
Cod liver oil capsule	800
Multivitamin tablet	800

Vitamin D

Severe Vitamin D deficiency causes rickets in children. Bone growth is reduced and the bones become soft and liable to bend.

In adults severe deficiency causes osteomalacia (bone pain and thinning) and is an important factor in osteoporosis and bone fracture.

Vitamin D helps the immune system and reduces the risk of **cancer.**

Moderate vitamin D deficiency in adults, causes bone and muscle pain. It causes muscle weakness especially around the upper legs which makes the person walk more slowly with a waddling gait, have difficulty in rising from a sitting position and be more liable to unsteadiness and falls. A recent meta-analysis has suggested that vitamin D supplements can lower the risk of falling by about 20%.

Low levels of vitamin D are associated with faster progression of

Osteoarthritis of the hip and knee.

Vitamin D deficiency has also been associated with an increased risk of hypertension, cardiovascular disease, diabetes mellitus (type 1 and 2), chronic pain, depression, dental problems, multiple sclerosis, mental health problems, infections and cancer.

Vitamin D is obtained by the body from two sources

- the effect of sunlight on the skin
- fat in the diet.

It is then metabolised in the liver to produce 25-hydroxyvitamin D. This substance is then transported to the kidney where it is converted into active vitamin D.

Recommended daily intake is 400iu (10mg) but this is difficult to obtain from the diet alone.

Food sources of Vitamin D

- Oily fish are the richest source. (400iu in 2.5 servings of tuna.)
- Dairy products and eggs. (400iu in 30 litre milk, 1Kg butter or 9 eggs.).
- Fortified cereals.

Vitamin D deficiency is common in vegetarians.

During the summer exposure of the face, and hands to 30 minutes of sunshine and therefore UVB radiation to the skin a day is enough to provide sufficient daily vitamin D in the form of D3 (cholecalciferol).

Adequate cholesterol in the skin is required to form vitamin D.

Vitamin D production is reduced in the winter and in elderly and dark skins. Sunscreens greater than factor 10 will block vitamin D production. Those who cover themselves for religious or cultural reasons are at risk.

"Vitamin D deficiency is becoming more common in developed countries. Mild vitamin D deficiency affects about 55% of adults in the UK. Marked vitamin D deficiency is present in about 15% of all adults in the UK but 30% of those over 65 years old and about 95% of otherwise healthy South Asian adults. People at risk include those who have inadequate exposure to sunshine such as housebound people, those in residential care, the elderly and certain ethnic populations such as Asian, African, Middle Eastern due to their clothing or dark skin."

Drugs and Therapeutics Bulletin. April 2006

Sub clinical low vitamin D is common among young girls. UK researchers assessed blood biochemistry and estimated sun exposure in 51 girls from an inner-city multi-ethnic school. They found 73% were vitamin D deficient and 17% severely deficient. Vitamin D concentration was related to the estimated duration of sunlight exposure and percentage of body surface area exposed. This was higher in white compared with non-white girls due to religious and cultural differences. There was no association with estimated vitamin D intake in the diet. The researchers warned that "deficiency of vitamin D in childhood and adolescence might impair the acquisition of peak bone mass at the end of skeletal growth and maturation." *(Arch Dis Child 2006)*

Vitamin E

Vitamin E, like other antioxidants, helps to prevent the build up of fatty plaques in our arteries and acts as an anticoagulant. It also has an important role in supporting the immune system.

Co-enzymeQ10 is required to recycle oxidised vitamin E.
Co-enzymeQ10 is reduced by statins.

The body can process food rich in the vitamin better than from supplements. Natural food sources are:

- vegetable oils e.g. olive and sunflower.
- Cod-liver and other fish oils
- Vegetables e.g. avocados and asparagus.
- Leafy green vegetables.
- Soyabeans and nuts
- Whole grains.

Recommended daily amount (RDA) is 30 iu. Toxic effects occur over 800 iu.

Vitamin K

Deficiency of vitamin K is rare as it is produced by intestinal bacteria in the gut and present in green leafy vegetables, potatoes, beans, tomatoes, meat and liver.

It may be deficient in the new born baby and cause haemorrhagic disease of the new born. Deficiency is more likely in premature babies and those that are not breastfed. The early breast milk (colostrum) is rich in vitamin K. Vitamin K is now given routinely to children at birth.

Deficiency of vitamin K in adults may be caused by warfarin therapy, malabsorption and prolonged antibiotic therapy.

Adequate vitamin K is important in preventing osteoporosis.

Researchers analysed data from seven trials including 1,000 patients who were given oral vitamin K supplements or placebo. All the trials showed that vitamin K supplements reduced the risk of hip fracture by around 77%, vertebral fracture by 60% and non vertebral fracture by 80%, compared with placebo. *(Arch Intern Med. 2006)*

Summary of Fat soluble Vitamins

Vitamin	Effect of Deficiency	Effect of Toxicity
A	Night blindness, dry eyes, xeropthalmia causing blindness, headaches. dry skin, acne, reduced resistance to infection and cancer. kidney stones	Hepatitis, birth defects, Osteoporosis
D	Rickets, osteomalacia, osteoporosis, bone pain, muscle weakness/spasm, cancer	Nausea, vomiting, headache, depression, calcification of arteries
E	Reduced resistance to infection, skin problems, irritability, reduced resistance to nerve and cardiovascular disease	Nausea, diarrhoea, weakness, palpitations
K	Excessive bleeding, osteoporosis	Thrombosis

Have adequate sunshine

Our ancestors had more sun exposure by working outdoors. Vitamin D deficiency did not become a problem until after the industrial revolution when a large number of people moved from the fields to the factory. Our indoor life leaves 50% of us depleted in vitamin D at certain times of the year.

Population studies show that, in America, the further south you go, the greater the sunshine and ultraviolet B doses and the lower the rates of cancer. Australian melanoma rates continue to rise even though sunscreen is widely used. Sun creams work better against UVB which promotes vitamin D production and less against UVA which is more harmful.

People with dark skins are at greater risk of vitamin D deficiency.

They have more melatonin in their skin which acts as a natural sunscreen and blocks vitamin D production.

Sunlight helps reduce depression. When sunlight enters the eye it stimulates the cells in the brain to produce more mood boosting serotonin. We produce about six times more serotonin in summer than we do in winter. This means we have less stress, more energy and lower levels of depression.

Vitamin D helps the absorption of calcium and is needed to develop healthy bones and teeth. Osteoporosis is less common in sunny countries.

Sunlight also reduces the risk of heart disease.If 7-dehydrocholesterol is not converted to vitamin D by sunlight, more cholesterol is present in the blood. In addition, sunshine causes vasodilatation, reducing blood pressure and improving circulation.

Vitamin D is involved in balancing insulin levels and reduces the risk of diabetes.

Sunlight seems to improve the immune system, lowering the risk of

autoimmune diseases such as rheumatoid arthritis.

Vitamin D and sunshine

U.S. research revealed that deaths from cancer including colon, ovarian and breast cancer are only half as high in sunny regions as in low sun areas

Prof. William Grant a retired Nasa scientist and director of the Sunlight, Nutrition and Health Research Centre in California thinks moderate exposure to sunshine does more good than harm.

Excessive exposure to the sun is thought to cost about 1,600 deaths a year in the UK from melanoma skin cancers. However insufficient exposure to the sun is thought to cause 25,000 deaths a year from cancer generally. *One sixth of all cancer deaths could be prevented if we sunned ourselves a little more.*

Prof. Grant and other scientists have established vitamin D deficiency as a key cause behind 17 different types of cancer including melanoma. Vitamin D helps abnormal cells to destroy themselves and if they don't then cancer may start.

Cancer research UK says:

- Skin cancer will double in the next 30 years due to excess sun exposure.
- People should avoid excess sun and burning.
- Stay in the shade between 11am and 3pm.
- Cover up with a T-shirt and use factor 15.
- Deliberate sun exposure is not good for health.

Prof. Grant says:

- Skin cancer is increasing because overuse of sun cream stops skin darkening and thickening to stop UVA penetration.
- Vitamin D deficiency is encouraging melanoma and skin cancers.
- People should avoid excess sun and burning.
- Expose your skin for short periods in the middle of the day when ultraviolet rays are strongest and vitamin D is produced fast.

Avoid excess sugar
Have a low GI carbohydrate diet

The human body is designed to obtain most of our calories and energy from carbohydrates. In primitive times humans ate complex carbohydrates such as vegetables, fruit, whole grain, beans and lentils.

Man learnt that most sweet plants were not poisonous. These were digested and glucose slowly released so that blood sugar levels never went very high. These foods also contained essential vitamins and minerals and the less digestible carbohydrates provided fibre.

Cultivation of grains and tubers such as potatoes provided an increase in carbohydrate to the diet on a regular basis.

Modern man discovered how to extract the sweetness but leave behind the nutrients and fibre to make processed sugar. The processed or refined simple sugars cause a much more rapid rise in blood sugar than the original complex carbohydrates and therefore have a higher glycaemic index.

High blood sugar levels are toxic and insulin is required to transport glucose from the blood into cells. High glycaemic index (G.I.) foods cause a strong insulin response. They provide bursts of energy followed quickly by a drop in blood sugar and hunger.

Frequent stimulation of the pancreas to produce insulin may decrease the sensitivity of cells in some people. The cells make fewer insulin receptors and become insulin resistant. Insulin resistance is associated with adult onset diabetes, raised blood lipids, stubborn obesity, high blood pressure, and cardiovascular disease.

Diabetes

Type 1 diabetes (insulin-dependent) occurs all over the world and in undernourished communities is the predominant type. It has been thought in the past to be an inherited problem but there is increasing evidence that it may be related to diet or infection. Early exposure to Cow's milk protein and hormones may be a factor.

Type 2 diabetes (non-insulin dependent) is closely linked to an excessive consumption of refined sugar and obesity. Genetic factors make it more likely to occur in certain groups. The risk is greater in those who have emigrated

BLOOD SUGAR AND INSULIN

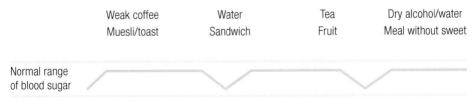

Poor diet (high GI)

| Sweet strong coffee | Cola | Cola | Sweet tea | Beer |
| Cornflakes | Chocolate bar | Hamburger and Chips | Cake | Meal with sweet |

High blood sugar

Insulin surge

Manic mood

Normal range of blood sugar

Low blood sugar

Irritable, poor concentration

Good diet (low GI)

| Weak coffee | Water | Tea | Dry alcohol/water |
| Muesli/toast | Sandwich | Fruit | Meal without sweet |

Normal range of blood sugar

No extremes of blood sugar, insulin or mood

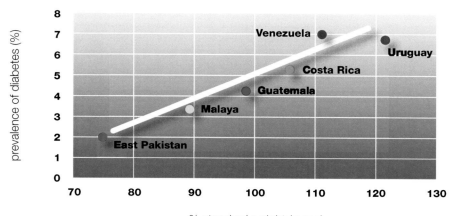

Diabetes and Obesity from ABC of nutrition – BMJ 1985

prevalence of diabetes (%) vs *% standard weight (mean)*

Diet and Diabetes

	Diabetes Prevalence	% of energy provided by:			
		Total Carbohydrate	Sugar	Protein	Fat
East Pakistan	2.0%	83	2	10	7
Malaya	3.3%	68	8	11	21
Guatemala	4.2%	73	10	12	15
Costa Rica	5.4%	69	17	11	21
Uruguay	6.9%	53	12	14	33
Venezuela	7.0%	62	7	14	24

Note increased incidence of diabetes with high fat/high protein as well as high sugar diet. Lower incidence in vegetarian countries and higher incidence in those countries with a higher intake of animal meat and dairy products.

to the west and developed a western diet after coming from a country where their ancestors had for thousands of previous years a largely vegetarian and low sugar diet. Obesity is a major factor especially if they develop predominantly central or abdominal obesity with a large waist circumference.

High fat intake as well as a high sugar intake is more likely to lead to diabetes than a high total carbohydrate diet. High total carbohydrate diet (mostly starch) and high fibre intakes are characteristic of peasant communities, in which type 2 diabetes is uncommon. They eat mainly low G.I.(glycaemic index) foods rather than the high G.I.foods and drinks that are common in affluent societies.

Low G.I.(gylcaemic index) sugars

- Fructose (G.I. = 19) found in all fruit and in honey. It is about 40% sweeter than ordinary sugar but provides about 40% fewer calories and causes less tooth decay. It absorbs water better than sugar so products containing fructose stay fresh for longer. Fructose is absorbed slowly. It has to be converted to glycogen in the liver before being converted to glucose.
- Lactose (milk sugar) (G.I. = 46) found in milk and dairy products. Less sweet than sugar. 80% of adults worldwide have a low level of lactase, the enzyme needed to break down lactose to glucose and galactose. They cannot tolerate an excess of milk or dairy products.

High G.I (glycaemic index) sugars

- Sugar (sucrose) (G.I. = 68) from sugar cane or sugar beet. Consists of equal amounts of glucose and fructose.
- Glucose (dextrose) (G.I. =100) found in some fruits and in honey. Needs no digestion, quickly absorbed and causes rapid rise in blood sugar and insulin levels.
- Maltose (malt sugar) (G.I. = 110) found in beer. It consists of two molecules of glucose chained together. (Wine contains fructose GI=19)

Sweet drinks are a major factor in many peoples high G.I. diet.

Britain's thirst		
	2006 Sales £m	**% change since 2001**
Cola	1217	+ 25%
Pure juices	1074	+ 65%
Water	643	+ 95%
Flavoured fizzy drinks	539	- 24%
Fruit drinks	529	+ 16%
Energy drinks	520	+ 174%
Squash	455	+ 10%
Lemonade	137	- 1%

Source Nielsen/Britvic.

Hypertonic drinks or "energy drinks" contain more than 10g of sugar a litre and inhibit fluid (water) absorption. They provide energy but very little fluid and increase thirst:
Lucozade energy. (17.9g sugar = 73 cal. per 100ml)
CocaCola (27g sugar+33mg sodium+23mg caffeine =97 cal per 100 ml)
Fanta Orange (35g sugar + 35mg sodium =111 cal per 100ml)

Isotonic drinks or "sports drinks" contain about 4 to 8g of sugar per litre and a small amount of salt. This provides some glucose for energy during exercise, but not so much that it prevents the absorption of fluid.:
Lucozade sports (6.4g sugar+50mg sodium+9mg potassium=28 cal per100ml)

Hypotonic drinks contain less than 4g of sugar a litre and help the absorption of fluid and rehydration. The effect is helped by the addition of more sodium (salt). Very little energy is supplied:
Dioralyte (1.8g sugar+235mg sodium+150mg potassium per 100ml)
Diet Coke (0.1mg sugar+ 28mg sodium+ 31mg caffeine = 1.0 cal per 100ml.
No sugar, stimulants to raise blood sugar, but no nutrients.

Sugar

The refining of sugar cane and sugar beet removes almost all minerals and nutrients. Nutrients such as zinc, chromium and molybdenum are required in minute quantities to make various enzymes including those involved in digestion. Sugar uses far more nutrients in its digestion than it supplies, so it tends to drain the body of important minerals.

World Health Organisation and Government guidelines are that, in adults, not more than 10% of calories should come from sugar. (excluding fructose and lactose.)

 10% = 50g = 200 cals. = 12 level teaspoons

A can of carbonated soft drink contains the equivalent of 8 to 10 teaspoons of sugar.

Low sugar food = up to 2g of sugar per 100g

High sugar food = over 10g of sugar per 100g

Sugar and Chromium

Chromium was only found to be an essential mineral in the 1950's and its importance for insulin was only noted in the 1970's. Chromium is part of the insulin receptor and improves insulin production and efficiency. It also helps reduce cholesterol levels, stimulates the synthesis of important proteins such as neurotransmitters and helps the immune system. Many people are deficient in chromium because the refining of sugar, rice and wheat removes almost all of the chromium together with other important nutrients.

People's sugar intake has increased dramatically over the last few years and this requires them to produce more insulin to suppress high blood sugar levels. A prolonged relative deficiency of chromium is an important factor in producing insulin resistance and diabetes. It may also cause depression. In many studies chromium supplements have helped control diabetes.

Good sources of chromium are whole grain cereals, cheese, eggs, brewer's yeast, spices, nuts, beans and meat (especially beef). Fruit and vegetables have very little and refined grain (white bread) almost none.

High GI diet

Sugary foods affect your immune system and reduce your resistance to infection. A white cell in normal blood can destroy 14 germs in one hour, but, if exposed to a high blood sugar, the white cell only destroys 2 germs in one hour. High sugar and insulin levels, by affecting the immune system increase the risk of infection and cancer.

A high GI diet decreases the amount of vitamin C that you absorb by 25%. This is because both glucose and vitamin C are competing for the same absorbing process and if blood sugars are high less vitamin C is taken into cells. Vitamin C is important in boosting the immune system and reduces the risk of cardiovascular disease by improving the health of the artery walls and reducing the stickiness of the blood. Research suggests that people with high vitamin C levels live up to six years longer than those with low levels.

Children and adults on high GI diets have been shown to be more likely to be lacking in zinc, iron, folate and calcium. This is because refined sugar and white refined bread have had almost all of their vitamins and minerals removed.

How to avoid or help diabetes

- Avoid obesity
- Avoid excess sugar in food and drinks.
- Avoid excess alcohol especially beer which contains the high GI sugar maltose.
- Avoid processed foods such as biscuits, cakes, snack bars which tend to be high in refined sugar and trans-fats. They are very low in chromium and cause the body to lose chromium when they raise the blood sugar.
- Avoid an excess of fried food and crisps which contain trans-fats.
- Have low GI carbohydrate as in wholegrain bread, pasta, vegetables and fruit.
- Have wholegrain bread and cereals which are low GI and provide fibre and essential nutrients such as chromium which helps insulin work and reduces insulin resistance. Chromium is also in meat, cheese and egg yolk. Fruit and vegetables have very little chromium and refined grain products such as white bread almost none. Smoking and excess caffeine can also deplete chromium.
- Have the spice cinnamon which increases the effect of insulin. It also lowers LDL cholesterol and is an antioxidant.
- Have oat bran which contains beta-glucan a nutrient which has a marked effect on reducing blood sugar and also LDL cholesterol. It is low G.I. and also provides fibre. Oat bran is present with oak flakes in cereals, porridge and oat cakes.

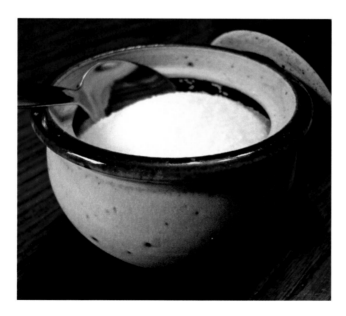

Avoid excess chocolate

Chocolate is made up of cocoa mass, cocoa butter and sugar to which milk, vanilla and other substances may be added.

The more cocoa mass the chocolate contains the better it is for your health.

- Dark plain chocolate contains 70% cocoa mass.
- Milk chocolate contains 20%.
- White chocolate contains 0%

Cocoa contains

- Flavonoid antioxidants.
- Phenylalanine is an important neurotransmitter which stimulates and reduces stress.
- Theobromine is a stimulant and cough suppressant.
- Anti-blood clotting factors which reduce the risk of thrombosis.
- Calcium, iron and potassium.
- The stimulants increase serotonin in the brain improving mood.

Although there is some health benefit in dark chocolate it must be remembered that milk chocolate is extremely high in calories, sugar and saturated fat. Most chocolate products have a high glycaemic index, causing blood sugar to rise quickly and stimulate high insulin levels. This may increase the risk of diabetes.

Chocolate bars are popular and promoted strongly at newsagents, motorway service stations and garages. The average Briton eats the equivalent of 154 bars of chocolate a year. The UK chocolate market was worth about £3.6 billion in 2004.

Chocolate bars are addictive, have poor nutritional value and a high content of sugar, saturated fat, trans- fats and calories. They increase the risk of obesity, diabetes and cardiovascular disease. I believe that, like cigarettes they should carry a health warning and advertising be banned.

Avoid obesity

Obese people have an increased risk of:

- High blood pressure.
- Coronary heart disease.
- Type 2 diabetes.
- Osteoarthritis, joint pain and joint replacement.
- Falls and fractures.
- Sleep disorders.
- Cancer especially of breast and bowel.
- In addition there are the psychological effects which may lead to low self-esteem and depression.

Obesity, size of the problem

In 2006

- 29% of men and 26% of women in the UK were obese (BMI over 30)
- In the US the obesity rate is now 55%.
- 15% of 15 year olds in the UK are obese.
- 10% of 5 year olds are obese.

There has been a 75% increase in obesity over the last 10 years.

Extreme obesity (BMI over 40) occurs in 3% of females and 1% of males. Extreme obesity has increased over the last 10 years by times three in females and by times five in males.

The proportion of overweight (BMI over 25) and obese (BMI over 30) people is about 50% in the UK and about 65% in the USA.

Why obesity is increasing

- More meals eaten outside the home which are higher in fat and sugar.
- Less cakes and biscuits eaten but more confectionary, snacks and

fizzy drinks.

- 'Super sizing'- Larger portion sizes.
- Excess of sugar which has no nutritional value (no minerals or vitamins) but provides a lot of calories.
- 50 – 100 calories each day above energy needs can result in weight gain of 5 to 10 lbs a year.
- Lack of exercise.

Potential benefits of 10Kg weight loss in 100Kg adult or 10% weight loss

- 10 mmHg fall in systolic blood pressure and 20mmHg fall In diastolic.
- 10% fall in total cholesterol (LDL fall of 15%. Triglycerides fall of 30%. HDL increase of 8 %.)
- 50% reduction in risk of diabetes (50% reduction in fasting glucose.)
- 20 – 25% reduction in total mortality.

One million fewer obese people in the population could lead to

- 15,000 fewer cases of coronary heart disease.
- 34,000 fewer cases of type 2 Diabetes.
- 99,000 fewer cases of Hypertension.

Why overweight?

- Calories in (Food) = Calories out (Exercise) - Weight steady.
- Calories in more than Calories out - Weight increases.
- Calories in less than Calories out. - Weight decreases.

Fat contains twice as many calories as carbohydrate or Protein.

Carbohydrate and protein = 4 calories per gram

Alcohol = 7 calories per gram

Fat = 9 calories per gram

To lose weight

No special diet is required. Just have smaller quantities of a varied and healthy diet containing plenty of fruit and vegetables.

Avoid an excess of sugar and fat. Avoid sweet drinks. This decreases your calorie intake.

Increase the amount of exercise. This increases the amount of calories you lose.

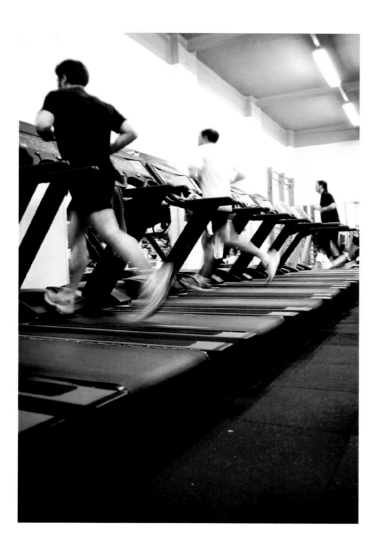

Exercise

In the past people were required to do a lot more exercise as an essential part of their lifestyle. Hunting and gathering food, then farming, required a lot more exercise than the modern industrial age with its many labour saving devices such as washing machines, telephones and cars.

A larger amount of food and calories were justified in the past and this was mainly provided by natural, mainly raw foods of good nutritional value.

Today there is less need for as much exercise and calories. Unfortunately food is more plentiful and cheaper but not as nutritious because of intensive farming and the refining of food.

Exercise is important to burn up any excess of calories provided in your diet. This prevents obesity. Exercise reduces aches and pains by stimulating the body's endorphins and also reduces anxiety and depression.

Moderate exercise taken daily has greater benefits than the occasional short burst of intense activity. Lifespan is increased by moderate exercise but decreased by very little or excessive exercise. Walking, swimming, dancing, cycling, or using stairs rather than lifts or escalators are better activities than a short visit to the gym.

> *"Exercise reduces LDL (the bad cholesterol) and raises HDL (the good cholesterol). It can lower the blood pressure and make the blood less likely to clot. 20 minutes of exercise three times a week can reduce the risk of coronary heart disease by up to 50%."*
>
> **(British Heart Foundation report 1994)**

Inactivity is as dangerous as being overweight, smoking 20 cigarettes a day, high blood pressure or high cholesterol.

Exercise and calories

Activity	Calories burnt per hour
Running	500
Swimming	430
Nordic walking	400
Cycling	280
Walking briskly	300
Strolling	100
House cleaning	100 to 150
Cooking	80
Shopping	100
Standing still	10
Watching TV	5

Figures based on average performance by 12 stone person.

On average slim people move about for an extra two hours a day, burning off an extra 350 calories. Over one year this equates to a weight loss of 2 to 3 stone.

A Kentucky Fried Chicken meal contains about 900 calories. To burn these off a person would have to walk six miles. A Pizza Hut Super Supreme pan pizza contains about 2,770 calories. Side order of garlic bread contains about 400 calories. To burn these off requires 21 miles on the treadmill which could take six hours at the gym. A burger meal (large burger, fries and cola) contains 1300 calories.

Normal daily average calorie intake is
2500 for men and 2000 for women

Have adequate fruit and vegetables

It is estimated that diet may contribute to the development of one third of all cancers. After stopping smoking, increasing fruit and vegetable consumption would do most to reduce cancer.

Benefits of fruit and vegetables

- Reduces the risk of cancer
- Reduces the risk of cardiovascular disease (e.g. heart attacks and strokes.)
- Lowers blood pressure
- Reduces the risk of cataracts and macular degeneration
- Reduces the severity of asthma.
- Reduces constipation.
- Helps reduce the risk or severity of diabetes.

The World Health Organization states that 85% of cancers in adults could be prevented if we include the equivalent of five portions of fruit and vegetables in our daily diet. The main reason is that most or some of these foods are eaten raw and are full of vitamins, minerals, phytochemicals, other anti-oxidants and fibre.

Eating more than five portions of fruit and vegetables a day reduces the risk of stroke by 26%. Eating between three and five portions a day reduces the risk by 11%. This was the result of pooled data from eight studies involving 257,000 participants in Europe, the US and Japan. comparing fruit and vegetable consumption and stroke incidence. (Researched by Dr Feng He of St Georges Hospital, London and published in the Lancet Jan. 2006.)

It was also noted that increased fruit and vegetable consumption would reduce other forms of cardiovascular disease and some cancers.

(The Times Jan. 2006)

Anti-cancer

Polish women's risk of breast cancer triples after they migrate to the USA, rising to the average American rate. This is thought to be associated with a reduction of cabbage in their diet. A study presented to the American Association for Cancer Research in 2005 showed women who ate four or more raw cabbage servings a week as adolescents are 70% less likely to develop breast cancer as adults. The Poles in their homeland are keen on cabbage which they tend to eat raw or lightly cooked. Sauerkraut and coleslaw are popular forms.

Cabbage contains anti-carcinogenic myrosinase enzymes and glucosinolates. These substances are reduced greatly by overcooking cabbage as tends to happen in the UK. In 1982 the National Research Council on Diet, Nutrition and cancer found "there is sufficient epidemiological evidence to suggest that consumption of cruciferous vegetables is associated with a reduction in cancer".

In 1992 a researcher at John Hopkins University discovered a compound in broccoli that prevented the development of tumours by 60% and reduced the size of tumours that did develop by 75%. Because of such reports, broccoli became one of the best-selling vegetables in the USA.

A recent meta-analysis of 87 studies confirmed that broccoli and other cruciferous vegetables significantly lower the risk of cancer. One study showed a 50% reduction by those eating two servings of half a cup a day.

Researchers at the Harvard School of Public Health USA studied 48,000 men over 10 years and found a gradually decreasing risk of bladder cancer

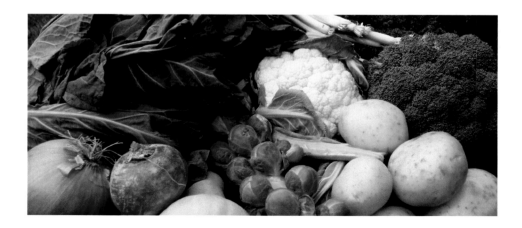

associated with an increasing consumption of green vegetables.

"The Mediterranean diet in many studies has been shown to reduce the risk of cancer. It has been found that oleic acid, the main fatty acid in olive oil, is as effective as Herceptin in killing the Her2/neu protein, a major factor in the growth of breast cancer tumours. When combined with Herceptin there is a reduction of 70% in Her2/neu levels in test tube experiments."

Prof. Javier Menendez and team at University of Chicago. USA. New Scientist Jan. 2005

"Women who consumed olive oil more than once a day were 25% less likely to develop breast cancer than were women who used olive oil once per day or less."

Trichopoulou etc journal of the National Cancer Institute. Jan.1995.

Other studies have shown a reduced risk of breast cancer with high intakes of fish or fish oil, folic acid, vitamins B6 and B12.

Most studies show a reduced risk with high levels of carotenoids present in fruit and vegetables. Glucarate a compound found in many fruit and vegetables improves the immune system and binds to carcinogens before safely excreting them. There is a lot of evidence that a high intake of fruits and vegetables is protective against most cancers. There are a number of possible factors that help:

Vitamin A (beta carotene)

Folic acid

Vitamin C

High fibre

Phyto-oestrogens such as isoflavonoids and lignans.

Other phytochemicals

Willett etc. American Journal of Clinical nutrition. May.1994.

Vegetarians

Vegetarians are 30% less likely to die of heart disease and 40% less likely to die of cancer.

(12 year study BMJ 1995)

A vegetarian diet is likely to contain more fibre and micro-nutrients and less saturated fat. Life span is increased only by a few years on average but their quality of life is often greater as they have less illness. Vegetarians who do not eat enough, such as the elderly, are more at risk of some vitamin and mineral deficiencies, in particular deficiencies of vitamin B12, vitamin D and iodine.

Vegetarians are at risk of having too much omega-6 and not enough omega-3 as no fish are eaten. Seaweed (kelp) is helpful in providing iodine if no fish are eaten. However it is easy to have excess which may cause the thyroid problems that you are trying to avoid.

Vegetarians have:

Less coronary and cerebrovascular disease.

Less hypertension

Less obesity

Less diabetes.

Less diverticular disease.

Less appendicitis.

Less constipation.

Less food poisoning.

Less hiatus hernias.

Less haemorrhoids.

Less varicose veins.

Less gallstones

Less kidney stones.

Less osteoporosis.

Less gout

Less cancer.

Have fresh whole foods rather than processed foods

Whole foods such as fruit and vegetables are very complex and contain many important nutrients, some of which we do not yet know about. This is why trials of individual vitamins are extremely difficult to evaluate and why whole foods are superior to vitamin and mineral supplements.

For example a substitute for spinach would have to contain the following but it would be impossible to duplicate the exact proportions which may provide an important synergistic effect:

- Vitamins A (beta-carotene) C, B1, B2, B6, E, K and folate.
- Co-enzyme Q10,
- Minerals calcium, iron, magnesium, manganese and zinc.
- Essential fatty acids omega 3 and omega 6.
- Phytonutrients lutein, zeaxanthin, glutathione, alpha lipoic acid.
- It also has chlorophyll, which is thought to have a powerful anti-cancer effect and other substances which are not known about.

Natural raw fruit and vegetables provide carbohydrate in a matrix that contains simple sugars, complex starches and fibre. This causes a slow rise in blood sugar and reduced insulin response as compared to refined and processed foods. The risk of diabetes is decreased.

Natural fruit and vegetables contain phytonutrients, vitamins, minerals and other nutrients many of which are destroyed by refining, processing or cooking.

Raw or lightly cooked fruit and vegetables are the most nutritious foods available.

Phytonutrients

There are more than a thousand known phytonutrients. They are present in all natural plants and are plentiful in fruits, beans, vegetables, whole grains and herbs. Many refined and processed foods contain none or very little.

They are not classified as essential nutrients but help protect against disease and degeneration.

Most phytonutrients act as antioxidants reducing the risk of cardiovascular disease and cancer, e.g. flavonoids (fruit), carotenoids (fruit,carrots.), polyphenols (tea, grapes), allyl sulphides (garlic, onions, leeks).

Many stimulate enzymes. e.g. indoles (cabbages), protease inhibitors (beans), terpenes (citrus fruit, cherries).

Some act like hormones. e.g. isoflavones (soya bean) imitate oestrogen and help to reduce menopausal symptoms and osteoporosis.

Some phytonutrients reduce DNA replication which helps prevent cancer. e.g. saponins in beans, capsaicin (hot peppers).

We will become more knowledgeable about phytonutrients in the future and many will be synthesised and promoted as supplements. The advantages of whole foods is that a large number of phytonutrients are present which are designed to work together. Whole foods rather than supplements would be cheaper and make life less confusing.

Green vegetables. e.g. broccoli, cabbage, brussels sprouts, kale, cauliflower, watercress, rocket.

Broccoli contains: -

Fibre

Low fat protein

Complex carbohydrates – low GI

Essential fatty acids – Omega-3 and 6.

Vitamins B6,C, E, K, beta-carotene, folate and CoQ10.

Minerals: calcium , magnesium and potassium.

Phytonutrients:

Sulphoraphane –antioxidant and anti-cancer.

Indoles – anti-cancer.

Lutein/zeaxanthin – carotenoid antioxidants that help prevent cataract and age-related macular degeneration.

The raw vegetables have more vitamin C, but cooking makes more carotenoids available. Broccoli and other "greens" are goitrogens and excess (over two cups) may reduce thyroid activity

Beans: also known as legumes or pulses. They include all beans, peas, lentils and peanuts. They are a good source of:

Fibre

Low-fat protein

Essential fatty acids (omega 3 and 6)

Complex carbohydrates

Vitamins - B including folate.

Minerals - Iron, potassium, magnesium.

Phytonutrients including phytoestrogens.

Beans are one of the most healthy and economical sources of protein.

One cup of lentils provides 17g protein and 0.75g fat. (Two ounces of lean sirloin steak has the same amount of protein but six times the amount of fat.)

Tomatoes: classified as vegetable although really a seed bearing fruit. They contain:

Fibre

Low fat protein

Complex carbohydrates

Vitamins A, B (thiamine, niacin, pyridoxine, pantothenic acid, Biotin and folate.) vitamins C, E

Minerals potassium, chromium, magnesium, manganese and zinc.

Phytonutrients. lutein, zeaxanthin, carotenoids, lycopene, phytoene and phytofluene

The yellow liquid surrounding the seeds has been found to have a powerful effect on reducing platelet stickiness and the risk of thrombosis. Tomatoes reduce the risk of cancer, cardiovascular disease, macular degeneration and skin sun damage.

Lycopene is a caratenoid and contributes to the red colour in tomatoes. It is also in watermelon and pink grapefruit. It is fat soluble and its actions are helped by vitamin E so eating it with fat such as olive oil or cheese helps. A pizza provides a good combination of tomato sauce and cheese. Lycopene is a powerful antioxidant that reduces the risk of cancer. It protects LDL cholesterol from oxidation reducing cardiovascular disease. It helps protect the skin from sun damage. Together with the other carotenoids, lutein and zeaxanthin it reduces the risk of macular degeneration. Lycopene is more available to the body from cooked tomatoes.

A Harvard medical school study in 1995 of 48.000 men found that those who ate ten or more servings of tomatoes a week reduced their risk of prostate cancer by 35% and their risk of aggressive tumours by 50%. In 1999 the same team showed that two servings of tomato sauce a week significantly reduced the risk of prostate cancer. The prostate contains a large amount of lycopene and this may be the main anti-cancer compound but other compounds may contribute. A synergistic effect involving several compounds may be important.

Berries: blueberries, cranberries, purple grapes, loganberries, raspberries, strawberries, currants, cherries, blackberries etc.
Berries are packed with nutrients which have a synergistic effect. They include:

Fibre (pectin a soluble fibre) helps bowel problems.

Low fat protein

Complex carbohydrates

Vitamins A (carotenoids) B2, B3, folate, C and E.

Minerals, potassium, magnesium, manganese and iron.

Phytonutrients - polyphenols and phytoestrogens

Salicylic acid which reduces the risk of thrombosis (equivalent to taking low dose aspirin.)

This is why raw grapes, grapefruit drinks and wine have for many thousands of years been considered nutritious and good for your health.

Soy: soya bean products include tofu, soya milk, soy nuts, tempeh, edamame and miso. Soy contains :

Fibre

Low fat (no cholesterol) high quality protein(all the essential amino acids)

(half cup of tofu provides 19g protein = 2 oz lean sirloin steak.)

Soybeans are 35% protein, fish is 22%, hamburger is 13%, milk is 3%.

Complex carbohydrates.

Omega-3 and omega-6 essential fatty acids

Vitamins E and folic acid.

Minerals: potassium, magnesium and selenium.

Phytonutrients including phytoestrogens .

Two of the isoflavines in soy – genistein and daidzein – reduce atherosclerosis and decrease the ability of tumours to grow new blood vessels and spread. They also decrease the growth of new blood vessels in the retina reducing the risk of visual loss in age-related macular degeneration.

In many studies a high intake of soya has been found to reduce cardiovascular disease, diabetes, age-related macular degeneration, osteoporosis, hormonal problems and cancer.

Women in Asia who consume diets high in soy have a four to six times less risk of breast cancer compared with American women who have little soy. This is thought to be due to the isoflavine genistein which acts like a weak oestrogen. It binds to sites on cell membranes competing with the more potent natural oestrogen and reducing its effect. In this way it helps prevent hormone dependant cancers of breast and prostate. It also helps menopausal symptoms and reduces the risk of osteoporosis.

Soy products allow people with lactose intolerance who cannot tolerate milk to have adequate calcium and protein. (Yogurt is another alternative.)

Cereals such as oats and wheat germ. Oats contain:

Fibre

Low fat protein

Complex carbohydrates (low G.I.)

Essential fatty acids (omega -6 and omega-3)

Vitamins: B1 (thiamine) B5 (pantothenic acid) E.

Minerals: magnesium, manganese, potassium, zinc,

copper, iron and selenium.

Phytonutrients : polyphenols, phytoestrogens, lignin's, etc.

Garlic: garlic lowers cholesterol and blood pressure. It reduces the tendency to blood clotting reducing risk of heart attacks and strokes. It helps the immune system fight infections. It has antiviral, antifungal and antibiotic properties. It reduces the risk of cancer.

Garlic and other 'allium' vegetables such as onions, leeks, chives and shallots are rich in sulphur containing amino acids that help make glutathione, a powerful antioxidant which reduces the risk of coronary heart disease and cancer. Homocysteine levels are reduced.

Tea: is an example of a beneficial herb. Herbs often contain valuable phytochemicals and other nutrients. A small amount of a variety of different herbs is advised.

Tea contains:

Flavonoids (antioxidant)

Fluoride (helps teeth and bones)

Caffeine (stimulant)

Tea contains more than 4,000 chemical compounds. It contains the same type of flavonoids as red wine and berries. Compounds in tea inhibit the formation of tumours and detoxify some carcinogens.

Drinking tea reduces the risk of cancer of the breast, prostate, lung oesophagus, stomach, pancreas, colon and bladder. Prostate cancer is fifteen times higher in the USA than in Asia and part of the reason may be the difference in tea consumption.

Tea consumption reduces the risk of cardiovascular disease especially if taken without milk. It lowers LDL cholesterol and homocysteine levels.

Tea drinkers were found to have arteries with less atherosclerosis than coffee drinkers. However coffee also has helpful phytonutrients which act as antioxidants.

A Harvard study showed a 44% lower risk of heart attack in people who drank at least one cup of tea daily.

The fluoride content of tea helps the health of teeth and bones.

Have wholemeal bread rather than white bread.

Bread is made by milling wheat seeds into flour. Bread was originally baked locally and had a short shelf life. Today flour comes from high-speed rolling mills that replaced slow traditional mills in the early 1800s. The faster and more efficient new mills generated more heat which converted the grain fats to oils and made them more easily oxidised. The flour became rancid and spoiled more quickly. The solution was to remove the fatty acids by removing the germ from the grain. To increase the efficiency of the milling process the outer layer (bran) of the grain was also removed. Millers could produce this new flour more cheaply than stone ground flour. It was more popular and it had a much longer life in storage. It could now be produced in large factories at long distances from the consumer.

Whole grains or wholemeal

A wholegrain may be wheat, barley, oats or any other cereal seed. It consists of three layers.

- The outer layer: the bran provides fibre, B vitamins, minerals, protein and phytochemicals.
- The middle layer: the endosperm provides carbohydrates, B vitamins and proteins.
- The inner layer: the germ provides Essential fatty acids, vitamins B and E and many phytochemicals.

The synergy of these three components gives an added effect.
For instance, vitamin B1 (thiamine) in the outer layer helps the metabolism of carbohydrate in the middle layer.

Whole grains

When grains are "refined" to make white flour or white rice the outer bran and the inner germ layers are removed. This removes most of the nutrients. The effect is a reduction in:

Fibre,

Vitamins B and E,

Minerals such as chromium, magnesium, manganese, molybdenum, phosphorus, selenium and silicon and zinc, (about 80% of magnesium, manganese and zinc are lost and about 98% of chromium is lost.)

Numerous phytochemicals which help enzyme and hormone actions and protect against cell damage which reduces the risk of cancer.

Essential fatty acids omega-3 and omega-6.

Nutrients	Wholemeal difference	Wholemeal bread (medium slice)	White bread (medium slice)
Kcals		74	78
Fibre (g)	4 times more	2.1	0.5
Sodium (mg)		205	191
Potassium (mg)	2 times more	83	36
Calcium (mg)		23	36
Magnesium (mg)	4 times more	28	7
Phosphorus (mg)	2 times more	72	28
Iron (mg)	2 times more	1.04	0.5
Zinc (mg)	3 times more	0.68	0.18
Selenium (mg)		13	10
B1 (mg)	2 times more	0.14	0.07
B2 (mg)		0.03	0.02
B6 (mg)		0.04	0.03
Folate (mcg)	2 times more	15	6

Adapted from What Are You Eating - Isabel Skypala.

People who eat whole grains have a reduced risk of twenty types of cancer according to a review of forty studies in 1998 and published in Nutrition and Cancer.

In a study of 34,000 post menopausal women in Iowa USA over nine years, those who ate a serving or more of wholegrain foods each day had a 16% lower mortality than those who rarely or never ate whole grains. Vitamin E intake from food has been inversely related to the risk of stroke. Whole grains and nuts are the two major food sources of vitamin E.

In the Nurses Health Study among the group that never smoked, an intake of two or three servings of whole grains a day was associated with a 50% reduction in strokes and a 30% reduction in coronary heart disease. The decreased risk of stoke may partly be due to reduction of blood pressure that occurs with a high fibre diet.

Sliced bread became available in the 1930's. By law, since 1956, the following have been added to white and brown bread.

Vitamins B1 (thiamine) and vitamin B3 (niacin).

Minerals Calcium and Iron.

Wholemeal bread already contains these nutrients and many more. Providing vitamin B3 (niacin) virtually eliminated the incidence of pellagra, a nutritional deficiency of vitamin B3 which causes dementia, dermatitis and diarrhoea. Providing vitamin B1 reduced beriberi which was a cause of heart failure. It is interesting to note that both vitamin B1 and B3 deficiency can cause psychosis and other severe mental health problems. White bread before 1956 may have been responsible for a great deal of mental illness including schizophrenia.

In 1956 chlorine dioxide was added to white bread. It bleaches, sterilizes and prevents rancidity. Chlorine also destroys any essential fatty acids and vitamin E that remain. Chlorine also destroys methionine an essential amino acid.

White bread

After refining, white flour consists mainly of fine particles of starch, a carbohydrate with a high glycaemic index. After eating white bread, blood sugars rise faster than with wholemeal bread. This increases the risk of insulin resistance and diabetes.

The risk of diabetes is also increased by the reduction in chromium, 90% of which is lost in the refining process of flour, rice and sugar.

Chromium reduces insulin resistance and increases the efficiency of insulin. Chromium also helps the synthesis of neurotransmitters such as serotonin reducing the risk of depression. In addition, It helps the immune system fight infection and reduces the risk of cancer.

The high added calcium content of white bread, and the fact that magnesium is almost totally removed in the refining process, means that there is a relative magnesium deficiency. The calcium/magnesium balance is important in preventing hypertension, osteoporosis and vitamin D deficiency.

The high calcium/low magnesium ratio is made worse by the addition of butter and cheese to the white bread in the popular cheese sandwich..

The development and popularity of white bread (70% of bread consumption) probably played a major part in the increase in diabetes, obesity, cardiovascular disorders, peptic ulcers, dental caries, osteoporosis, mental health disorders and cancer in the 20th century.

Bread

In the traditional process, which allows for slow fermentation, the correct amount of acidity is produced to break down the gluten and yeast. However, bakers are under pressure to produce cheap, fast bread with a long shelf -life. Now, high speed mixers are used which make the process so fast that the gluten and yeast are not broken down and are more likely to cause intolerance or a bloated feeling when eaten.

Bread is mainly flour, yeast and water. "Improvers" are designed to enhance volume, taste, structure and shelf-life. They include enzymes, emulsifiers and stabilisers. Salt and trans- fats are often added as improvers. The future for white bread may lie with lower sodium, higher fibre, and improved mineral and vitamin content but if possible more people should switch from white to wholemeal bread.

Avoid vitamin deficiency

Adequate vitamins are usually supplied by a good balanced diet.

If you have a good diet and add supplements such as cod-liver oil and multivitamins you may be getting an excess of fat soluble vitamins: too much vitamin A may increase the risk of osteoporosis, and too much vitamin D may increase calcification of arteries and tendons.

There is very little risk from an excess of water soluble vitamins such as B and C which are not stored in the body and so do not accumulate.

Fat soluble vitamins A, D, E and K are provided by plants, meat fat, dairy products, and eggs.

Sunshine is an important source of vitamin D.

Vitamin B is provided by whole grain bread and cereal, nuts and seeds.

Vitamin C is provided by fruit and vegetables.

The most common vitamin deficiencies are of folic acid and B12.

Folate (folic Acid) or vitamin B9

Most people are folate deficient. It is a water soluble B vitamin which is excreted within a few hours.

Five servings of fruit or vegetables are required to guarantee a recommended dose of 400mcg a day. An average diet provides 200mcg a day.

Overcooking destroys 90% of folate in food. 80% of old people in hospitals are folate deficient. 40% of teenage girls and 50% of men are folate deficient.

Folic acid deficiency is common in mental health problems.

Folic acid is in green leafy vegetables, root vegetables, mushrooms, fruits, nuts, pulses, wholemeal bread and cereal.

Pregnant women are advised to have 400 mcg daily from early pregnancy. Ideally there should be no folate deficiency in either partner at the time of conception.

In 1970 Dr Richard Smithalls reported a link between insufficient folate and spina bifida. It took 20 years before his work was taken seriously. In 1992 the US and UK Governments recommended for the first time ever a nutritional supplement. Pregnant women were advised to take 400mcg of folate daily, an amount not easily achieved by diet alone.

Folic acid supplementation in early pregnancy reduces both first occurrences and recurrences of neural tube defects by about 70%. Women with repeated miscarriages in a Dutch study were nearly twice as likely to have MTHFR genetic defect and high homocysteine levels which would have been helped by folic acid supplements.

Folate supplements prior to and throughout pregnancy reduce the risk of birth defects, miscarriages, premature birth and low birth weight. Vitamin B12, vitamin B6, zinc, omega-3 and magnesium supplements also lower homocysteine levels and reduce the risk of miscarriage. They may also reduce the risk of Down's syndrome and childhood epilepsy.

US law in 1996 required supplement of 140mcg folate to 100g of flour, rice, pasta, cornmeal and other grain products. Since the introduction of folic acid fortification of flour in the US a 20% fall in the incidence of neural tube defects has been noted, as well as a fall in incidence of myocardial infarcts and strokes.

In Canada fortifying flour with folic acid has cut the number of neural tube defects such as spina bifida by more than three quarters.

There is no fortification in Europe yet.

In 2000 the UK committee on medical aspects of food and nutrition policy recommended folate supplements for the UK. Further recommendations to the health minister were made in September 2006. The Agency committee estimates that about 800 pregnancies are affected by neural tube defects in the UK each year. An unknown number of miscarriages also result.

The main concern is a possible risk that fortification of flour would disguise Vitamin B12 deficiency signs and symptoms. Unrecognised B12 deficiency could lead to irreversible neurological damage.

Women with lower levels of folic acid are more likely to have low-birth weight babies according to a study at the University of Newcastle 2005. A Study of 998 expectant mothers showed a strong link between folic acid levels in the blood and birth weight. For each unit change in the folic acid level the baby's weight increased by 14%.

Expectant mothers who smoked were more likely to have lower levels of folic acid which may explain why they tend to have small babies. About 7% of all newborn babies are of low birth weight (less than 2.4Kg or 5lbs 8oz) and they have a 50% chance of having a severely disabling condition as a result.

Vitamin B12

Cyanocobalamin (oral) or Hydroxocobalamin (injectable)

Vitamin B12 deficiency is common.

Vitamin B12 is produced by bacteria present in dirt which is then eaten by herbivores and produces B12 in the large bowel. These bacteria are present on the surface of the leaves and roots of plants but then destroyed by the sterilization of plants with chlorine or other chemicals before being sold to the public. Carnivores obtain their B12 by eating herbivores. Unlike other B vitamins, B12 is stored particularly in the liver of animals and fish. It is present in fish, eggs, milk, cheese, meat and liver but is not present in most plants.

Deficiency commonly occurs in strict vegans. Vegans can obtain B12 from Spirulina, an aquatic plant green algae, or miso, which is made by fermenting Soy, rice or grains with yeast.

Metformin is a drug taken for diabetes which can cause B12 deficiency.

Deficiency may also occur if there is a lack of intrinsic factor in the stomach, which is essential for the absorption of B12. This occurs in pernicious anaemia which is a common auto immune disorder. An amino acid, homocysteine, requires B12 and folate to metabolize into neurotransmitters and antioxidants.

Deficiency of B12 causes:

High homocysteine levels.

A smooth sore tongue,

Anaemia.

Nerve degeneration causing tingling and pains mainly in the legs. Mental deterioration with poor memory, depression, psychosis and dementia.

Treatment is by a change of diet, oral supplements or injections of Vitamin B12.

Keep your homocysteine level down

Since the early 1990s, evidence has slowly increased that elevated levels of homocysteine are associated with an increased risk of birth defects, miscarriages, low birth weight, low IQ, atherosclerosis with cardiovascular disease, rapid ageing, cancer and poor mental health including depression and dementia.

Some people (10 to 15%) have a genetic defect causing a reduction in the enzyme which metabolises homocysteine (more common in Caucasian and Japanese). Homocysteine levels are about 25% higher than average in these people and they have a 20% excess risk of a heart attack or stroke.

Studies show high homocysteine levels (above 12 units) in adult's acts as an oxidant and increase the risk of cardiovascular disease as much as high cholesterol or smoking.

An excess of cysteine made from homocysteine reduces the absorption of insulin by cells reducing glucose tolerance.

Homocysteine levels tend to be higher in vegans and vegetarians than in meat eaters, unless they have B12 supplements. This is surprising as there is much less methionine in plants than animals. Any lack of B12 makes the recycling of homocysteine to methionine more difficult.

A trial in Chile in 1999 observed that folate levels were higher in vegetarians than meat eaters. However, their homocysteine levels were also higher. Adding B12 supplements lowered the vegetarians homocysteine levels from about 13 mmols to 8 mmols per litre. Average vegan homocysteine levels are about 15 mmol per litre. However their cholesterol levels are lower than average.

Vitamin B12 and folic acid are required in the methylation of homocysteine into methionine and the synthesis of SAMe (S-adenosyl methionine). SAMe is involved in numerous methylation reactions involving proteins and phospholipids which repair DNA and form the neurotransmitters. It is also involved in the synthesis of coenzyme-Q10 and other amino acids including creatine.

A defect in the methylation process is thought to cause the neurological and

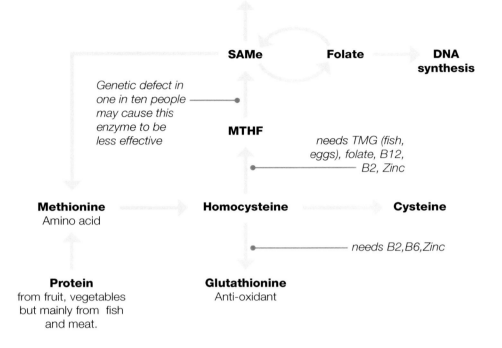

Neurotransmitters: SEROTONIN, MELATONIN, TRYPTAMINE, ADRENALINE, NORADRENALINE, DOPAMINE, ACETYLCHOLINE.

SAMe   Folate   **DNA synthesis**

Genetic defect in one in ten people may cause this enzyme to be less effective

MTHF

needs TMG (fish, eggs), folate, B12, B2, Zinc

Methionine
Amino acid

Homocysteine

Cysteine

needs B2,B6,Zinc

Protein
from fruit, vegetables but mainly from fish and meat.

Glutathionine
Anti-oxidant

psychiatric disturbances seen with vitamin B12 and folic acid deficiency. This defect in methylation reduces the production of methionine and increases homocysteine levels.

The neurotoxic effects of homocysteine may be partly responsible for the effects of vitamin B12 and folic acid deficiency.

Vitamin B12 and folic acid deficiency both cause similar problems including anaemia, depression, dementia, and a demyelinating myelopathy.

About 75% of mentally-ill people have a methylation disorder. Methylation problems are present in most schizoid and schizophrenic cases and are often helped by dietary advice and supplements.

Folic acid supplements have been shown to reduce homocysteine levels. It has been estimated that 800micrograms daily of folic acid would be sufficient to attain the required reduction in homocysteine levels. This would cause a 20% reduction in cardiovascular disease if given to all those over 55 years old.

B12 and B6 supplements also lower homocysteine levels.

High homocysteine levels have a prothrombotic effect and reducing these levels would reduce the incidence of strokes and deep vein thrombosis as well as heart attacks. Trials using folic acid, B12 and B6 supplements to lower homocysteine levels have shown a reduction in the symptoms of heart disease and evidence of a reduction in the rate of progression of atherosclerosis.

Supplements of folic acid, B12, B6 together with B3 (niacin), essential fatty acids (omega-3 and omega-6) and zinc have helped many cases of autism, attention deficit, depression, schizophrenia and psychoses.

A trial of supplementation in pregnancy of 4 mg of folic acid a day reduced the incidence of neural tube defects such as spina bifida by about 70%. A trial of supplementation in pregnancy of 0.8 mg of folic acid and 0.4 mg of B12 reduced neural defects by 100%.

Homocystinuria is a rare genetic disorder where children lack the enzyme which converts homocysteine, a naturally occurring but potentially toxic substance, into cystathionine, a harmless substance, and then to glutathione, an important anti-oxidant, or SAMe, a natural anti-depressant.

Children with homocystinuria have very high levels of homocysteine in their blood (over 100 units- normal under 12) and, unless treated, die at a young age of heart attacks and strokes despite having normal cholesterol levels. Post mortems show severe atherosclerosis.

How to reduce homocysteine blood levels:

- Avoid a high animal protein diet so that the supply of methionine is reduced.
- Have adequate folate and other B vitamins especially B6 (pyridoxine) and B2 (riboflavin) (wheat germ, green vegetables, nuts, avocados, seeds, liver, kidneys, eggs, milk and cheese.)
- Have adequate vitamin B12 (fish, shellfish, seaweed, meat especially organ meat such as liver, dairy products such as milk, cheese and eggs.)
- Avoid an excess of coffee, smoking and alcohol (especially spirits) which increase homocysteine.
- Have adequate minerals especially zinc (shellfish, fish, nuts, peas, turnips, whole wheat grain, oats, rye, eggs).

Avoid mineral deficiency

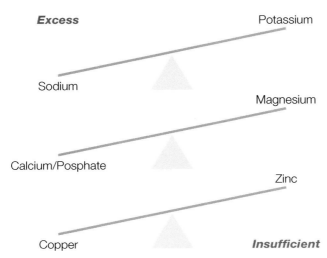

Mineral Balance

Excess — Potassium — Sodium

Magnesium — Calcium/Posphate

Zinc — Copper — Insufficient

The body tries to keep various minerals in balance.

At present most people have an excess of sodium, calcium, phosphate and copper.

The sodium/potassium and calcium/magnesium balances have been dealt with in the sections on salt and dairy products.

Zinc/Copper balance

The zinc/copper ratio is very important for good health. A high calcium or phosphorus intake may reduce the body zinc. A high intake of milk and dairy products, containing high levels of calcium and phosphorus, and cola drinks, which have a high phosphorus content, will therefore reduce zinc levels.

 High copper content of blood depresses zinc absorption from the intestine. High zinc intakes can reduce copper absorption.

An increase in the copper/zinc dietary ratio from the normal 1 to 4 causes increased homocysteine and blood cholesterol leading to atherosclerosis.

Modern houses have copper pipes and softened water will absorb some copper. It is important therefore that occupants have a high zinc intake or filter the water.

Copper deficiency is rare but zinc deficiency is very common. Over 50% of adults have less than the recommended amount, and an even greater percentage of pregnant women, children and the elderly are deficient. Vegetarians tend to have a low zinc intake as absorption from plants is poor. Meat eaters should get enough zinc but the levels in white meat are much less than those in dark meat. A high dairy or cola intake reduces zinc absorption.

Zinc

Zinc is one of the most important trace elements in the diet. After iron, it is the most common trace element in the body. It is necessary for over 200 enzyme activities. It is the principal protector of the immune system and regulates genetic information. It is required for protein and DNA synthesis playing a vital role in growth and cell division, (both copper and zinc are involved with the transcription of genes.)

Zinc is involved with the metabolism of protein, carbohydrates and lipids. Insulin is made from amino acids and zinc. It is an important antioxidant. It is important for metabolism in the ovaries and testes which affect fertility. There are high levels in the prostate and semen so that men require a higher intake than women.

Vegetarians require more as there is lower absorption of zinc from plants. Alcoholics, cigarette smokers, diabetics and people with chronic colitis or renal disease all require a higher intake of zinc.

Zinc helps prevent macular degeneration, infertility, lack of libido, anorexia, hair loss, acne. It maintains the sense of taste, smell and vision, helps wound healing, improves appetite and growth and reduces lethargy and fatigue.

Deficiency has been associated with an increased risk of dyslexia in children. Zinc is needed for the synthesis of the calming neurotransmitter GABA in the brain. Zinc deficiency is associated with irritability, anxiety and violent behaviour.

Zinc is found in fish, oysters, poultry, meat, egg yolk, mushrooms, nuts, beans, seeds and wheat germ.

Copper

Copper is an essential component of many enzymes, including those involved in antioxidant defence, connective tissue formation and neurological function.

Copper and iron are both required for haemoglobin synthesis and the prevention of anaemia.

Copper is present in nearly all foods. Very high levels of copper are found in liver. High levels are also found in shellfish, nuts and wholegrain cereals. It is also in mushrooms and chocolate.

Milk and dairy products are among the poorest sources of copper. Difference in soil levels and the effect of flour milling can affect the amount of copper in cereals and bread.

In the UK drinking water has been a valuable source of dietary copper due to leaching from domestic pipes especially when the water is softened. This will decline if the copper pipes are replaced by plastic alternatives or the tap water is filtered.

Copper promotes the production of stimulants dopamine and noradrenalin. (zinc is required in the synthesis of the calming neurotransmitter GABA.) High copper and low zinc levels may cause irritability, anxiety and violent behaviour. They have been associated with autism, post-natal depression and paranoid schizophrenia.

High copper and low selenium levels have been associated with an increased risk of atherosclerosis.

Iron

Iron is essential for making the haemoglobin in red cells which carries oxygen in the blood.

Deficiency causes people to feel weak, tired and short of breath.

Meat, liver and fish are rich in iron. Vegetarians can get adequate amounts from beans, peas, green leafy vegetables, whole grains and dried fruits such as raisins and apricots.

Calcium

Calcium is important in providing healthy bones and avoiding osteoporosis. It is an important constituent of the blood, extra cellular and intracellular fluids and helps prevent vascular constriction and hypertension. A high calcium, low magnesium diet causes constriction of blood vessels and a raised blood pressure.

A high caffeine consumption reduces calcium absorption.

Calcium is present in green leafy vegetables, nuts, beans, potatoes, oranges and bananas. Milk and cheese are high in calcium but the high protein content reduces the amount available.

Meat, fish, eggs and wheat, which are high in protein and low in calcium, all have a negative effect on calcium levels as they increase calcium excretion.

Low blood calcium levels cause an increase in parathyroid hormone which by increasing the production of vitamin D helps calcium absorption. A high calcium diet reduces the production of vitamin D.

Calcium excretion and loss by the body are increased by:

A high salt intake

A high protein intake

A low potassium intake.

On a typical western high protein, high sodium diet about 1000 mg of calcium is required daily. On a vegetarian high potassium low protein intake about 200 mg is sufficient.

Phosphorus

After calcium, phosphorus is the most abundant mineral in the body.

It is important, together with calcium, for the mineralization and health of bones and teeth. The absorption of phosphorus, as well as calcium, is under the control of the parathyroid hormone and vitamin D.

Phosphorus helps protect cell membranes and helps the function of vitamin B and many hormones and enzymes. It helps form DNA. It is necessary for the conversion of carbohydrates, protein and fat into energy. It combines with fats and proteins to form phospholipids which are vital in the brain and nervous system to transmit messages to muscles, glands and organs.

Phosphorus is present in most foods and deficiency is rare. It is particularly high in high protein foods such as fish, meat and dairy products. Cow's milk contains over six times the amount of phosphorus than human breast milk and over four times as much calcium. Processing the cow's milk reduces the calcium and increases the phosphorus which can cause a relative calcium deficiency. A relative hypocalcaemia in infants can increase the risk of convulsions.

Many popular soft drinks, including colas, have high phosphate content. Processed meats and other foods may have phosphate additives.

A high phosphate intake increases calcium excretion and the risk of poor bone health and osteoporosis.

Magnesium

Magnesium is essential for every biochemical process in our bodies, including metabolism and the synthesis of nucleic acids and protein. It is required in over 300 enzyme reactions:

- It helps the synthesis of DNA, cell growth and reproduction.
- It has an important role in immune function.
- It helps control neuronal activity, cardiac excitability, muscular contraction, vasomotor tone and blood pressure.
- It is necessary to prevent the calcification of soft tissue.
- Together with vitamin B6, it can dissolve calcium phosphate kidney stones.
- It has a protective effect on the arterial lining.
- It promotes the absorption of other minerals including calcium, phosphorous, sodium and potassium.

- It helps the utilisation of vitamin B, C and E.

Deficiency is associated with:

- Atherosclerosis, arrhythmias, heart attacks, strokes.
- Abnormal clotting (thrombosis)
- Depression and fatigue.
- Migraine
- Hypertension (20% of elderly have low magnesium)
- Pre-eclampsia in pregnancy.
- Diabetes-type 2 (40% have low magnesium).
- Osteoporosis
- Cancer.

Numerous studies have shown that magnesium deficiency can be a major factor in the causation of cardiovascular disease. Magnesium deficiency leads to an increased risk of hypertension, arrhythmias and myocardial infarcts.

Geographic regions low in soil and water magnesium have increased cardiovascular morbidity and mortality. Higher magnesium levels in hard water and mineral water are thought to be the reason that sudden cardiac death and myocardial infarcts are less likely in hard water than soft water areas.

Magnesium deficiency can cause a prolonged QT effect on the ECG (electrocardiogram) which can be responsible for blackouts or sudden death especially after extreme exercise. Supplementation of magnesium and potassium has been used successfully to treat and reduce arrhythmias.

Most people are deficient in magnesium. Diets provide about 200mg while recommended daily allowance is 300mg.

Symptoms of deficiency: muscle tremors or spasm, high blood pressure, irregular heartbeat, muscle weakness, constipation, insomnia, anxiety, depression, hyperactivity, convulsions, confusion and poor appetite.

Magnesium is found in fish, brown rice, fruits, spinach and other vegetables, nuts and seeds. It makes up part of chlorophyll and so is in all green plants.

An excess of milk and cheese may cause a relative magnesium deficiency.

Selenium

Selenium is a trace element that is an essential co-factor in the production of certain antioxidants such as glutathione and thyroid hormone. It plays an important part in the body's immune system reducing the risk of infections and cancers. In particular it appears to decrease the risk of prostate, bowel and breast cancer. It is important in the health of the eyes and skin. It helps to detoxify various toxins including alcohol. It helps produce healthy sperm.

Deficiency can cause muscle weakness, cardiomyopathy, goitre and hypothyroidism, miscarriage and infertility. Together with iodine and manganese deficiency, it can cause joint cartilage atrophy and degeneration (osteoarthritis). Marked deficiency is uncommon, but occurs where the soil is deficient in selenium and only locally produced food is eaten. This occurs in parts of Asia, Africa and North America.

Selenium is high in organ meats such as Liver and Kidney. Also in nuts, in particular, Brazil nuts (three of which can provide your daily requirement if they have come from selenium rich soil). Lesser quantities are in muscle meat, eggs, shellfish, fish, onions, tomatoes, broccoli, wheat-germ, corn and soya beans.

Wholegrain cereals and bread are a useful source of selenium depending on whether they are grown in selenium rich soil. In the UK, bread was an important source when flour was imported from the selenium rich prairies of North America. Now European flour is used and selenium levels in bread have fallen. This is believed to have played a major part in the fall of selenium intakes in the UK from an average of about 60mcg a day in the 1980's to about 40mcg today.

Recommended intake is over 60mcg a day.

In the UK, selenium intake is mainly from meat and eggs (40%), Cereals (20%).dairy products (15%) and fish (15%). Fruit and vegetables are low in selenium. Vegetarians are at risk of deficiency if they have cereals and bread low in selenium. However, they can compensate by eating nuts especially Brazil nuts.

In Finland selenium is added to fertilizers to increase the soil content.

Manganese

Manganese is important for many enzyme reactions.

Deficiency is common as it is not well absorbed.

Manganese is important for insulin production. Diabetics are often deficient.

It is also important in forming mucopolysaccharides in cartilage and deficiency may increase the risk of osteoarthritis.

It is important for brain health. Deficiency has been associated with an increased risk of Parkinson's disease and schizophrenia.

Manganese is in tea, fruit, nuts, seeds and whole grains.

Fluoride

Epidemiological studies have shown a definite relationship between the fluoride content of drinking water and the incidence of dental cavities. Levels of 1.0 to 1.5 p.p.m. are associated with minimum cavities and no mottling. Where there is a low level of natural fluoride in the water, the incidence of dental cavities is increased.

Fluoridation of water supplies to maintain a level of 1.0 to 1.2 p.p.m. is carried out in many parts of the world. Evidence shows no harmful effects and an average reduction of 60% in prevalence of cavities in permanent teeth of children.

Bone density studies in USA showed less osteoporosis in areas with high fluoride intake. Also, surprisingly, there was less calcification of the aorta.

In the UK, only 10% of the population, about six million people, receive fluoridated water, mainly in the Midlands and North-east. About 170 million Americans live in areas with fluoridated water.

Iodine

Iodine is an essential trace element mineral but its importance justifies its own section.

Have adequate iodine

The thyroid hormones determine our rate of metabolism. A deficiency slows down metabolism causing a reduction in physical and mental abilities. The thyroid hormones are formed by a combination of an amino acid, Tyrosine, and Iodine, an essential trace mineral.

Tyrosine is obtained from chicken, turkey, nuts, seeds, avocados, soya, bananas and dairy products. Tyrosine can also be made from another amino acid, phenylalanine, which is present in similar foods, and, additionally, in green leafy plants, whole grains and fish.

Iodine deficiency causes a lack of thyroxine (hypothyroidism)

Iodine is present in fish and seaweed. There is very little in fruit and vegetables and this is dependant on the soil content.

Essential fatty acids play an important role in thyroxine production. Vitamins A, B2, B3, B6, C and E are required for the synthesis of thyroxine. Minerals copper, selenium and zinc are also essential.

People who have a high cereal, high vegetable diet may reduce their absorption of iodine, together with other minerals, because of the high phytic acid or other goitrogen content. Phytic acid is present in most plants, and high in raw green vegetables and whole meal bread. It can combine with minerals to form phytates that are stable in the digestive system and so cannot be absorbed. Minerals affected include iodine, calcium, iron and zinc. Goitrogens are largely destroyed by cooking. Problems may occur if minerals are not obtained from other sources such as fish, meat, dairy products and seaweed.

Thyroid disease: the size of the problem

Over one in a hundred women in the UK will develop an under active thyroid. This is called hypothyroidism and is ten times more common in women than men. Sub-clinical borderline deficiency is extremely common. About one third of hypothyroid cases are thought to be due to auto-immune disease and the cause is unknown. A reaction to the thyroid hormone in dairy products is a possibility. Nutritional factors especially iodine deficiency are important and probably grossly underestimated.

Swelling of the thyroid gland is the most visible sign of iodine deficiency and hypothyroidism, but iodine deficiency and hypothyroidism may be a serious problem before reaching this stage.

Iodine is abundant in the oceans and the main foods that contain iodine are fish and seaweed such as kelp. Mountainous areas where there has been marked erosion have soil that is short of iodine as the original ocean bed is no longer present.

There is very little iodine in fruit and vegetables and the amount is dependant on the soil content of iodine. Fruit, vegetables, cereals and meat contain small amounts. (2 to 5 mcg per 100g compared to 30 to 600mcg per 100g in fish and 3000mcg per g in dried kelp.)

Recommended daily intake of iodine is 200mcg.

Excess of iodine (over 600mcg) may cause hyperthyroidism or hypothyroidism and this could easily happen if an excess of seaweed food such as kelp was taken on a regular basis.

Hypothyroidism is more common in vegetarians and people who do not eat fish or seaweed, or who drink milk.

Iodine content:

Seaweed (1 g dried)	=	3000 mcg
Cod (3 oz)	=	99 mcg
Iodized salt (I g)	=	77 mcg
Potato (1)	=	63 mcg
Cows milk (I cup)	=	56 mcg
Shrimp (3oz)	=	35 mcg
Egg (1)	=	29 mcg

In the US table salt has had iodine added since 1924. This dramatically reduced the incidence of goitre and hypothyroidism. For many years iodine has also been added to salt in Switzerland, Yugoslavia, New Zealand and some South American countries but not the UK. In Australia, the UK and some other European countries, iodine is added to animal feed.

Since 1990 there have been a number of projects to introduce iodized salt and vegetable cooking oil into populations in Africa, Asia and Europe. People in hot countries require more salt as they lose salt in sweat. However, excessive salt intake should not be encouraged because of the increased risk of hypertension. Efforts should be made to iodize the hidden salt in processed foods or encourage alternative sources of iodine such as fish or seaweed.

In the UK iodine is not added to salt on a compulsory basis but iodized salt is available. Iodine is added to animal feed so that milk becomes a good source of iodine in the winter but less so in the summer when the cows eat mainly grass.

Since the 1980's there has been routine testing at birth for hypothyroidism of every child as part of a heel prick test. 1 in 3,500 to 1 in 4,000 infants are found to be hypothyroid and treated with thyroxine to prevent cretinism. The problem is twice as common in girls.

Iodine deficiency

It is estimated that iodine deficiency causes a 10 to 15% reduction in a populations IQ capability. It causes mental retardation and cretinism. The virtual elimination of iodine deficiency was identified as the highest health priority for children at the 1990 World Summit for Children organised by the World Health Organization and UNICEF.

In 1993 The Progress of Nations reported that lack of iodine was affecting the mental and physical development of approximately 50 million children, condemning tens of millions to mental retardation and causing an estimated 100,000 children a year to be born as cretins. The solution – iodizing all salt supplies –had been available for decades. The world health organisation estimates that about two billion people, including 285 million school aged children, are still iodine deficient.

New England J Med 2006

One in 10 women in the UK have thyroid problems after giving birth. Their symptoms of tiredness and depression are often put down to postnatal depression. Researchers in a Dublin Hospital took urine samples from 54 women in early pregnancy. Urinary iodine excretion values suggestive of iodine deficiency were observed in 55% of those tested in summer and in 23% in winter. The researchers noted: "Adequate maternal thyroid hormone production is crucial for the proper neuropsychological development of the foetus. The findings are a cause of concern which, if confirmed by a more comprehensive investigation, may indicate the need for iodine prophylaxis." (Irish Journal of Medical Science 2006) In summer, milk comes from cows that feed on grass. The soil, and therefore grass, in most of Ireland is deficient in iodine. In winter, a greater variety of foods, some with iodine supplements, are given to the cows.

Education of pregnant mothers especially vegetarians in regard to optimal nutrition can be seen to be important but ideally this education should start in school so that both parents but especially girls are having a good diet before the onset of pregnancy.

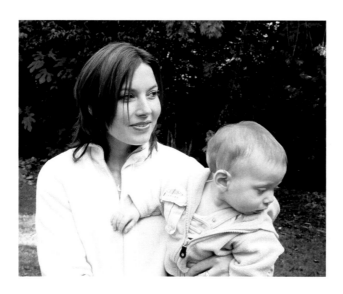

Have nuts and seeds

Nuts provide protein, carbohydrate, fat, vitamins and minerals. Fat in nuts is the healthier mono-unsaturated fat (like olive oil), which lowers LDL cholesterol and has heart protective effects.

Nuts, especially walnuts, are rich in essential fatty acids such as Omega-3, which has an anticoagulant and other beneficial effects.

Nuts provide one of the richest food sources of vitamin E which has anti-oxidant and anti-inflammatory properties. A high intake of vitamin E reduces the risk of type 2 diabetes and heart disease.

Nuts are a good source of iron, zinc, selenium, magnesium and potassium. Brazil nuts are a rich source of selenium and linked with a reduced risk of breast and prostate cancer, (study at University of Illinois). Low umbilical cord selenium is associated with an increased risk of childhood asthma (Avon UK study). Children in the bottom 20% of prenatal selenium exposure were more than three times as likely to develop asthma as those in the top 20%. Adequate selenium may reduce the risk of osteoarthritis.

Seeds, like nuts, contain all the essential nutrients for their particular plant. They are packed with nutritious vitamins, minerals and phytochemicals. They contain a balance of carbohydrate, protein and essential fatty acids, together with fibre. If eaten raw, none of the nutrients are lost by cooking.

Almond nuts contain:

Vitamin E : anti-ageing and anti-oxidant

Monounsaturated and essential fats.

Protein and fibre.

Low G.I. carbohydrate.

Magnesium: keeps arteries healthy and prevents arrhythmias.

Potassium: lowers blood pressure.

Phytochemicals.

Five major US studies have found that people who regularly eat nuts have a lower risk of heart disease. People who included almonds as part of their low calorie diet lost more weight, more body fat and had a bigger decrease in their waistline and blood pressure than another group on a low-fat, high–carbohydrate diet.

Walnuts Contain:

Protein

Amino acid Arginine (natural vasodilator)

Omega-3 fatty acids (anti-coagulant)

Vitamins B6, E. folate (reduce homocysteine)

Plant sterols (reduce cholesterol)

Polyphenols (antioxidant , anti-cancer, anti-inflammatory).

Minerals potassium, copper and magnesium (lower BP, anti-arrhythmic)

Fibre, (reduces insulin).

Nuts are low in saturated fat but high in monounsaturated and polyunsaturated fats. Polyunsaturated fat lowers blood cholesterol about twice as much as saturated fat increases it. As with other nuts, walnuts reduce the risk of cardiovascular disease, dementia and cancer.

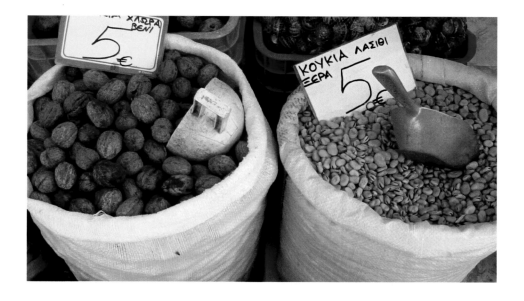

Have adequate fibre

Fibre is the part of plant food that the body cannot digest. Complex carbohydrates from plants are rich in fibre and starch.

Soluble fibre can bind with bile to reduce cholesterol. It slows the digestion and absorption of carbohydrates helping to stabilise blood sugar and reduce the risk of diabetes.

Insoluble fibre absorbs water in the large intestine and causes the stools to be larger and softer. This decreases the time that food travels through the intestines resulting in less exposure of the bowel wall to toxins and carcinogens. Fibre makes stools more acidic which reduces bacterial destruction and the production of possible carcinogens in the colon.

Processed food contains little or no fibre.

Dietary fibre

- Protects: against coronary heart disease.
- Lowers: post meal glucose and insulin levels,
  LDL (bad) cholesterol and blood pressure
- Increases: HDL (good) cholesterol
- Provides: B vitamins so homocysteine is reduced.

A fibre rich/low refined carbohydrate diet reduces :

Obesity and diabetes

Heart disease and hypertension.

Constipation, varicose veins, haemorrhoids,

Gallstones, appendicitis, hiatus hernia

Diverticulosis and bowel cancer.

Denis Burkitt (1911–1993)

Denis Burkitt made an enormous contribution to our awareness of the importance of fibre. While a surgeon in Uganda, Denis Burkitt noted that the Africans had a remarkably reduced incidence of bowel problems, obesity, diabetes, coronary heart disease and cancer. He noted the Africans' greater fibre intake, and that they produced a much larger quantity of soft faeces. He hypothesised that a major cause of Western disease was the consumption of refined carbohydrates with its low fibre content. In 1966 he came to London and, working for the Medical Research Council, launched a worldwide crusade to increase our consumption of vegetable and fruit fibre.

Dennis Burkitt's quotes.

"In Africa, treating people who live largely off the land on vegetables they grow, I hardly ever saw cases of many of the most common diseases in the United States and England - including coronary heart disease, adult onset diabetes, varicose veins, obesity, diverticulitis, appendicitis, gallstones, dental cavities, haemorrhoids, hiatal hernias and constipation. Western diets are so low on bulk and so dense in calories, that our intestines just don't pass enough volume to remain healthy."

"America is a constipated nation. If you pass small stools you have to have large hospitals."

"Diseases can rarely be eliminated through early diagnosis or good treatment, but prevention can eliminate disease."

"The only way we are going to reduce disease, is to go backward to the diets and lifestyles of our ancestors."

"Gall-stones is a disease of modern Western culture. It is estimated that a third of a million gall-bladders are removed annually in America. More is spent in the United States on taking out gall-stones than the total expenditure on preventive and curative health care in the whole continent of Africa. Yet it is largely a preventable disease.

In 20 years of surgery in Africa, I had to remove exactly one gallstone."

Fibre intake

Rural Africans eat about 55 grams of dietary fibre a day. In UK, average intake is 15 grams. Africans have the lowest incidence of bowel problems such as constipation, haemorrhoids, appendicitis, diverticulitis, colitis and bowel cancer. Africans also have a reduced incidence of obesity, diabetes and cardiovascular disease.

- Fibre - Recommended Daily Amount. (RDA) = 30g daily
- Medium slice of wholemeal bread contains about 2.6g fibre.
- Five portions of fruit or vegetables contain about 24g fibre.

Soluble fibre (e.g. hemicellulose, pectin, gums)

Dissolves in water. Helps lower cholesterol and regulate blood sugar.

In fruits, vegetables, wholegrain cereals and bread, beans, peas, seeds and herbs.

Insoluble fibre (e.g. cellulose, lignin's)

Absorbs water causing softer bulkier motion. Low calorie.

In fruits, vegetables, wholegrain cereals and bread, seeds and nuts.

Low fibre.

Potatoes – chips and crisps. white rice, white bread, porridge, lettuce, cucumber, tomatoes.

No fibre

Sugar, milk and dairy products- cheese and butter, eggs, meat and fish.

Bread: It's a great way to go

A study in Australia selected three towns.

- They promoted an increased consumption of wholemeal bread in the elderly with a slogan " Bread: it's a great way to go"
- There was a campaign by local doctors, the media and advertising.
- Also a reduction in the price of wholemeal bread.
- The campaign resulted in a 60% increase in bread sales and a 60% fall in laxative sales.

Most people on a western diet have inadequate fibre.

£43 million was spent on prescribed laxatives in the UK in 2004.

Have adequate water

Our bodies are about 70% water. Water provides the fluid for our blood, and digestive juices and helps lubricate joints and eyes. Loss of water though skin sweat, the lungs, mouth nose and sinuses and faeces helps to remove toxins and regulate temperature.

Dehydration causes tiredness, weakness, headaches, poor concentration and dry wrinkled skin. You can lose water and salt as sweat with exercise. Excessive vomiting causes water and mainly sodium loss. Excessive diarrhoea causes water and mainly potassium loss. There is risk of electrolyte imbalance if large quantities of water only are given as replacement. Having electrolyte replacement sachets may help. A slightly salty drink such as soup may replace sodium. Fruit juice is a good source of potassium.

Hydration in children

Under hydration in children may cause fatigue, poor concentration, irritability, constipation, urine infections, bedwetting and kidney stones. Children need water to convert food to energy quickly and efficiently. If deprived of it, their physical and mental responses rapidly slow down.

Just 5% dehydration (not enough to feel thirsty) can reduce your ability to concentrate by up to 20%.

Children up to five years old should drink six to eight cups of water, about 1.5 litres, a day; those up to ten years, about 1.75 litres; and older children and adults, about 2 litres a day.

When children are well hydrated they do not crave food and are therefore less likely to become obese.

A Tunbridge Wells school survey found that pupils drinking only water showed a nine fold increase in concentration levels compared with when they drank fizzy drinks. Sugar, additives and caffeine cause hyperactivity and poor concentration.

As can be seen in the section on avoiding an excess of sugar, there is an increase in consumption of nutritious pure fruit drinks, mainly by adults, but children still favour hypertonic drinks full of sugar and caffeine. The energy drinks, in particular, provide an excess of calories, increasing the risk of obesity and diabetes. The high GI sugar, caffeine and other additives can cause poor concentration, irritability, anxiety and depression. Drinking only hypertonic drinks without water can cause dehydration. The "diet" drinks have far less calories, but, because of the additional sweetener additives, may be more likely to cause mental health problems.

Tap water

Tap water is supplied by surface water from reservoirs, lakes and rivers and ground water from underground caves. A number of pollutants can enter the water supply. These may originate from acid rain, industrial waste, pesticides, fertilizers, and chemical waste. The pollutants are largely removed at water treatment centres.

Bacteria in the water are destroyed by chlorination, but chlorine itself is toxic and an oxidant which increases the risk of atherosclerosis and cardiovascular disease. For this reason, tap water is best not taken in large amounts unless filtered. A jug filter reduces about 75% of chlorine, copper, mercury and aluminium which is beneficial, but also calcium, magnesium and fluoride which is not beneficial. Boiling water removes the chlorine by evaporation.

People living in a chalk or limestone area have 'hard' water unless it is softened by the water company. This is often done to please the customers, as softened water does not fur up the water pipes and kettle. It is also easier to wash clothes and your body with, as it mixes with soap and 'lathers' more easily.

People living in a granite area have 'soft' water, which is acidic. Soft, acidic water is more corrosive to the water pipes it passes through and may lead to increased levels of copper, lead and cadmium. (Most modern water pipes are copper). Especially in houses with new copper pipes, the soft acid water encourages leaching of copper into the water. This may be beneficial in moderation, but may cause anxiety and poor mental health in excess, especially if inadequate amounts of zinc are consumed. Copper sulphate is sometimes used in reservoirs to reduce green algae.

Soft water is more acid and may increase the risk of osteoporosis, cardiovascular disease and hypertension. Softening water to reduce the furring up of pipes and kettle should not be done too enthusiastically.

Hard water contains more calcium and minerals from chalk or limestone. This decreases the risk of cardiovascular disease and hypertension. The water is more alkaline which reduces the risk of osteoporosis.

Mineral Water

Bottled mineral water originates from natural springs. It contains varying amounts of minerals such as calcium, magnesium, potassium, sodium and sulphate. Its main advantage is that it does not contain chlorine.

The high mineral content in some mineral waters may make it unsuitable for children, and people with high blood pressure should avoid those with a high sodium content.

Mineral water can be a useful source of essential minerals such as magnesium and calcium.

There is some concern that if plastic containers containing water are left in hot sunshine some of the plastic toxins may seep into the water.

Some of these toxins can upset hormone balance.

Drinks summary

Keep well hydrated by regular intake of water.

- Milk is a good source of protein, calcium and vitamin D, but intake should be limited because of the high animal fat, protein and hormone content. There is less fat and hormones in skimmed milk. Soya milk is a good substitute to have with cereals, but is not usually tolerable with tea and coffee.
- Coffee and tea contain antioxidants which reduce the risk of cancer. However, both contain caffeine, an excess of which causes anxiety and stress. Tea also contains fluoride (good for teeth and bones).
- Tea, coffee and alcohol have a mild diuretic effect which means that less water is retained by the body compared to drinking water.
- High sugar content makes a drink hypertonic and tends to dehydrate.
- High caffeine intake from an excess of coffee, tea or cola drinks may

cause anxiety and palpitations. This can be aggravated by insufficient hydration if no separate water is taken.

- Studies have suggested that a small daily intake of alcohol -especially of red wine - is beneficial and may reduce heart disease.
- Real fruit juice is nutritious and a good source of Vitamin C.
- Fizzy drinks are seldom nutritious and full of sugar. This increases the risk of obesity and diabetes.
- The artificial sweeteners in diet drinks carry health risks if consumed in excess.
- Mineral water has more minerals and less chlorine.
- Tap water is best filtered or boiled to remove chlorine.

Avoid excess alcohol

Evidence suggests that moderate levels of alcohol consumption exert a protective effect against coronary heart disease and reduce mortality. All types of alcohol are beneficial if taken in moderation.

Alcohol raises HDL (good cholesterol) and is a vasodilator. It reduces homocysteine levels possibly by providing vitamin B. The main benefit is from drinking small amounts on a regular basis (one to three units daily).

Excess alcohol has a toxic effect on the heart and liver. Large excess, e.g. 30 to 40 units a week, may cause cardiomyopathy and atrial fibrillation. Binge drinking (over 8 units) causes dehydration and an increased risk of myocardial infarct and stroke. A single binge episode of drinking increases the likelihood of accidental or deliberate self harm, hypoglycaemia, convulsions and stroke.

Study of 16,000 people in Copenhagen starting in 1970s. Moderate alcohol consumption was not associated with atrial fibrillation. But men drinking more than 35 alcohol units a week were 45% more likely to be suffering from atrial fibrillation.

Circulation 2005

Some people lack the enzyme that metabolizes alcohol and can only cope with small amounts, or get side effects more easily. About half of Japanese people have a deficiency of this enzyme. A deficiency is also more common among the American Indians, Australian Aborigines and Eskimos.

Beer

Beer contains malted barley, hops and yeast. It has many B vitamins and the minerals magnesium and chromium. Maltose, the sugar in beer, is very rapidly absorbed (G.I. =110) whereas, fructose, the sugar in wine, is slowly absorbed (G.I. = 19). Beer is therefore more likely to promote insulin resistance, obesity and diabetes. Substances in beer and other forms of alcohol boost tryptophan and serotonin levels. In moderation this improves our mood and promotes sleep. These substances also boost the anti-inflammatory hormones and reduce pain.

The average beer is only a third of the alcohol strength of the average wine. Beer, like other forms of alcohol in moderation, raises the good cholesterol (HDL), reduces platelet stickiness and fibrinogen. The risk of cardiovascular disease is reduced.

A study in Australia of 3,000 people in their 70s found that those who drank one or two beers a day had a 20% lower risk of dying of heart disease than those who were teetotal or drank to excess.

Drinking beer in moderation reduces the incidence of kidney stones. It also reduces the incidence of diabetes and osteoporosis. However, drinking to excess increases the incidence of diabetes and osteoporosis.

Wine

Wine contains a rich mix of cardio-protective nutrients.

Salicylates have an anti- platelet aggregation effect. This is the equivalent of taking low dose aspirin.

Ethanol causes vasodilatation and a slight reduction in blood pressure.

Flavonoids are antioxidants. They raise HDL and inhibit LDL oxidation in the plasma reducing the risk of thrombosis and atherosclerosis.

Red wines have the highest flavonoid content.

The French habit of drinking a glass or two of red wine with most meals may be a major reason for the low rate of coronary heart disease in France. (Other possible factors include more raw fruit and vegetables, local whole grain bread and mineral water).

The level of polyphenols in red wine is 20 to 50 times higher than white wine. This is due to the incorporation of the grape skins in the fermenting process. The polyphenols in grape skins are known to prevent the oxidation of LDL cholesterol thus reducing the risk of atherosclerosis and cardiovascular disease. There is also a reduced risk of dementia, cataracts and age-related macular degeneration.

The addition of 'friendly' bacteria in the fermenting process acts like a probiotic and reduces bowel problems.

If alcohol is to be avoided, similar benefits are available from purple grape juice, pomegranate juice, cranberry juice or prune juice. Dried berries contain similar nutrients but have less vitamin C and there may be a higher contamination with pesticides and fungicides.

Excess Alcohol

Excess alcohol consumption may lead to physical and mental problems.

- Physical: poor appetite, malnutrition, peptic ulcers. Excess alcohol and poor diet lead to deficiency of vitamin B such as thiamine and minerals calcium, magnesium and zinc. Liver damage and possible liver failure, impotence, poor memory and co-ordination. Damage to the liver may impair its ability to store fat soluble vitamins A,D,E and K and to metabolise protein. Cardiomyopathy and atrial fibrillation may be caused.
- Mental: Irritability, mood swings, depression, risk of job loss because of sickness, lateness and absenteeism. Memory loss and depression cause poor performance, safety concerns and bad behaviour or poor discipline. Risk of accident at home, work or with car is increased. Risk of marital and family problems or divorce is increased. Financial problems due to cost of alcohol, loss of job and divorce.

Recommended upper limits:

> Men: 3 to 4 units daily or 21 units a week.
> Women: 2 to 3 units daily or 14 units a week.

1 unit	= Half a pint of beer or cider.
	= One small glass of wine (125 ml of 9%). The average glass contains 2 units.
	= One measure of spirits.
Two pints of beer	= 400 calories

Alcohol abuse accounts for 70% of liver cirrhosis deaths which have risen nine-fold in young people since 1970. It also causes 150,000 hospital admissions a year and up to one third of all hospital casualty attendances.

Alcohol summary

- **Moderate amount reduces**:
  Cardiovascular disease.
  Dementia.
  Cataracts
  Gallstones
  Osteoporosis

- Lifespan is increased.

- Wine particularly red wine seems better than spirits or beer.

- **Excess causes**:
  Liver failure
  Pancreatitis
  Gastritis/peptic ulcer
  Oesophageal varices
  Malnutrition
  Peripheral neuropathy
  Impotence
  Infertility
  Foetal abnormalities
  Cancer
  Depression
  Dementia
  Osteoporosis
  Accidental or deliberate injury
  Hypertension and stroke
  Heart disease e.g. cardiomyopathy and atrial fibrillation
  Social problems – loss of job, financial problems, marital problems.

Avoid excess of additives

As with medicines, the greatest profits in the food industry are made if a new compound is found or created. It is then synthesised and the method patented. Because of this there are well over 700 synthetic flavour compounds. It is enormously difficult to know whether any side effects are due to one of numerous ingredients in the chemical cocktail of many processed foods.

The side effects of the older preservative additives in processed food have gradually been established by independent scientists.

- Salt excess: hypertension.
- Sugar excess: obesity, diabetes.
- Saturated fat excess: obesity, cardiovascular disease, cancer.
- Trans-fats excess: cardiovascular disease, inflammation, depression, cancer.
- Nitrites excess: methaemoglobinaemia, cancer, chronic obstructive pulmonary disease.
- Phosphates excess: hypocalcaemia, hypo magnesia, osteoporosis, attention deficit disorder.

"Because of the high consumption of processed foods it has been estimated that the average person in the UK and other industrialised countries will eat more than 4 Kilogram's of additives every year. The impact of this situation is still controversial as Governments have appeared reluctant to fund, conduct or publish rigorously controlled studies examining the effects of additives"

"Feeding Minds" Mental Health Foundation 2006

Additives

Additives are added to all sorts of processed foods to make them tastier, juicier, smoother, sweeter, more colourful and longer-lasting. All additives must be approved, and an Acceptable Daily Intake (ADI) given. 'E' number indicates that it is approved for use in Europe.

Preservatives:

Sodium benzoate (E211) may affect children's behaviour.

Sulphites (E220 to 227) including sulphur dioxide used in wine, beer and dried fruit can trigger asthma attacks.

Flavour enhancers:

Monosodium glutamate (E621) may cause headaches, chest pain, anxiety, flushing and numbness. In rare cases it may aggravate epilepsy.

Sweeteners:

Aspartame (E951), acesulfame K, and saccharin are sweeter than sugar and low in calories. Aspartame has been linked to neurological problems including headaches and dizziness, but the evidence was reviewed in 2002 and the conclusion was that it was safe.

Cyclamate (E952) was banned 30 years ago because of a possible link with cancer but ban lifted in UK in 1990s after further studies.

Sorbitol can accumulate and cause cell swelling. This is aggravated by high glucose levels as in diabetics and high galactose levels as in people on a high dairy diet. Diabetic like side effects may harm the kidney, nerves and eyes. Glaucoma may be made worse.

Antioxidants:

Vitamin C (ascorbic acid or E300) is added to foods that contain fats or oils to stop them going off or changing colour.

Emulsifiers:

These help mix ingredients that would normally separate, such as oil and water.

Stabilisers:

These prevent ingredients from separating again.

Gelling agents and thickeners:

Additives such as pectin(E440) and xanthan gum are used to make food smoother or to add bulk.

Colourings:

Beetroot juice (E162), the natural colouring annatto (E160b) can cause reactions in some people.

Colourings Tartrazine(E102), sunset yellow FCF(E110), carmoisine (E122), ponceau 4R (E124) and preservative sodium benzoate(E211) have been linked with hyperactivity and changes in children's behaviour by a recent Government study.

Some coal tar and azo dyes are still used but are gradually being reduced because of their known carcinogenic effect.

The body can cope with a small amount of toxins but an excess could be harmful. To avoid an excess of additives, try to avoid an excess of processed foods and have as much in the way of fresh whole foods as possible.

Avoid toxins and carcinogens

DNA damage

DNA damage is a normal event and it has been estimated that the DNA in a single human cell is damaged 10,000 times a day. This may occur when harmful by-products of natural chemical reactions are produced and when DNA is copied.

The ability of the body to repair DNA is shown by people who were exposed to huge doses of radiation at Hiroshima and Chernobyl and survived, and the unexpected finding that radiologists and nuclear shipyard workers live just as long, if not longer, than their colleagues.

Our ability to repair DNA becomes less efficient with age.

Excessive DNA damage may cause foetal abnormalities in pregnancy and an increased risk of cardiovascular disease and cancer.

DNA damage is more likely to happen if a person has inadequate antioxidants in their diet to cope with exposure to the numerous oxidants in the modern age which are potential carcinogens. Each living cell requires a mixture of anti-oxidants to protect it from damage by the oxidants. Inadequate defence or excessive attack can damage various parts of the cell. Our bodies produce many antioxidants on their own, but antioxidants in food are very important.

Fruit and vegetables are the best source of antioxidants as most antioxidants in meat are destroyed by cooking.

Damage to cells by unopposed oxidants may increase the risk of :

Osteoarthritis and osteoporosis

Atherosclerosis (furring up of arteries)

Cataracts, glaucoma and macular degeneration.

Dementia.

Eczema and asthma

Bowel disorders such as peptic ulcers and colitis.

Auto-immune disorders and infection.

Cancer by damage to the nuclear DNA.

Cancer

Oxidants (Potential carcinogens)

Cancer - the Battle

Oxidants	verses	Anti-Oxidants

⟵――――――――――――――――――――⟶

Oxidants	Anti-Oxidants
Toxins	Vitamins
Pollution	Minerals
Carcinogens	Phytonutrients
Radiation	Hormones
Excess Hormones	

- Tobacco smoke
- Petrochemical compounds e.g. diesel and petrol fumes, some food dyes.
- Some cosmetic dyes and other ingredients.
- Pesticide and insecticide residues.
- Mould on nuts and grains.
- Preservative nitrates in bacon, hot dogs, ham, salami.
- Smoked fish or meat.
- Charred meat.
- Malachite green: widely used in fish farming industry to control parasitic and fungal infections, (banned within Europe in 2002 because of research linking it to cancer in humans.)
- Acrylamide is a toxin linked to cancer and nerve damage. (More common in food cooked to high temperature, e.g. bread crusts, toast, chips, crisps and biscuits).
- Fats heated to high temperatures - 200.C or over
- Excess saturated fat
- Excess hormone levels.
- Excess alcohol.

- X-rays and solar radiation
- Infection with viruses, bacteria and fungi
- Inherited factors

Cancer may occur when carcinogen load overwhelms body's defences. Antioxidants in diet have a protective effect against toxic oxidants.

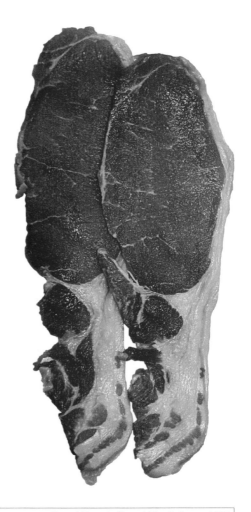

Avoid smoking

Cigarettes contain a chemical cocktail of more than 4000 different ingredients, including 43 known carcinogens and over 400 other toxins. With each inhalation a smoker receives small doses of carbon monoxide, arsenic, cyanide, DDT, nitrobenzene, formaldehyde, methanol, naphthalene and toluene, amongst other substances.

Cigarettes contain nicotine which is a stimulant. The nicotine is addictive and encourages the inhalation in cigarettes of many toxins and oxidants. These increase the risk of:

- Atherosclerosis causing cardiovascular disease and increasing the risk of heart attack, stroke and dementia.
- Chronic lung disease with recurrent bronchitis, chronic obstructive pulmonary disease (C.O.P.D.) and emphysema.
- Age related macular degeneration reducing vision.
- Premature ageing of skin with sagging and increased wrinkles.
- Cancer
- Smoking reduces a man's life expectancy by over 5 years and a woman's by over 6 years (Life expectancy is 81 years for men and 84 years for women.)
- At any age up to 80, the chances of dying in the next year are almost doubled by being a smoker according to Life Insurance company figures (2005).

Smoking and heart disease

Cigarette smoking increases the risk of atherosclerosis. Lipid soluble components of cigarette smoke may be absorbed and injure the artery walls. To prevent oxidation and atherosclerosis, antioxidants such as vitamin C and vitamin E are depleted. Smokers therefore require a higher intake of antioxidants to prevent atherosclerosis.

Cigarette smoke increases the tendency for blood to clot and the nicotine in tobacco constricts the arteries. Smokers have higher levels of plasma fibrinogen and have higher blood pressures. LDL cholesterol levels are high and HDL cholesterol levels low.

Smokers tend to have poor appetites. They tend to have:

- More fat (butter, chips, fried food and meat)
- More tea, coffee and alcohol which dehydrate. The excess of stimulants increases anxiety and the risk of depression.
- Less fruit and vegetables providing important antioxidants such as vitamin C.
- Less cereals and wholemeal bread providing antioxidants such as vitamin E and essential fatty acids.
- Dietary fibre and protein intake are also lower in smokers.

Smoking and eye disease

Smoking causes age related macular degeneration of the eyes to develop 10 years earlier than in non smokers. It is estimated that smoking causes or contributes to about 20% of blindness in people over 50 years old.

Research published in British Journal of Ophthalmology (2005) suggests that smoking may double your risk of age-related macular degeneration. This is the most common cause of blindness in the UK.

Smoking facts

- Men who smoke more than 20 cigarettes daily increase their risk of dying from a heart attack three fold.
- Women who combine smoking with oral contraception increase their risk of a heart attack and/or stroke by ten times.
- Infants born to women who smoke are small and frail.
- Men who smoke produce inferior sperm.
- Within a year of stopping smoking, the risk of a fatal heart attack drops by about half. After three smoke-free years, the risk falls to that of a non-smoker.
- The percentage of people smoking in the UK has reduced from over 50% in 1974 to below 30% in 2004.
- About 20% of 15 year olds smoke
- Cancer research UK estimates that tobacco has killed more than 6.3 million people across the UK during the last 50 years.

Have adequate sleep

A survey of more than a million Americans in 1960 showed an average time slept as 8 to 9 hours. In 2000 it had fallen to 7 hours. Our ancestors before fire and light was invented went to sleep when it became dark and only got up when it was light.

The stress hormone cortisol normally peaks in the body at midday and then falls until its lowest level is at the time you go to bed. Research has shown that sleep-deprivation causes a rise in cortisol levels. In young fit men, restricted to four hours of sleep a night for six days, their fall in cortisol level was six times slower than normal. The level of the hormone leptin also decreased by about 20%. Elevated cortisol and low leptin levels promote appetite and obesity.

Young children require 9 to 11 hours sleep. Staying up late to watch television may be a factor in childhood obesity.

A study published in 2004 found that those who slept nine hours or more had a significantly lower body mass than those who slept five hours or less.

Sleep deprivation reduces your efficiency at work and makes mistakes more likely. Chronic sleep deprivation is a major factor in the cause of work burnout and depression. Falling asleep at the wheel of a motor car is a major cause of car accidents and deaths.

Sleep

During the day, the brain is stimulated by the neurotransmitters adrenaline, noradrenalin and dopamine. Stimulation is also caused by stress which increases cortisol. The stimulation is decreased by another neurotransmitter gamma aminobutyric acid (GABA) which starts to reduce adrenaline and noradrenalin production and increase serotonin production in the evening as light fades. The effect of GABA is increased by sleeping tablets and tranquillizers and decreased by stimulants such as caffeine and nicotine.

Alcohol causes an initial increase in GABA producing a calming effect, but, about two hours later, there is a rebound reduction in GABA producing a stimulating effect which may cause anxiety, depression and difficulty in sleeping.

In the evening serotonin levels increase and, as it gets darker, serotonin produces another neurotransmitter called melatonin. Melatonin is essential for a good nights sleep and waking early is often a sign of serotonin, and therefore melatonin, deficiency.

"How much sleep we have affects our IQ, our suicide risk, our chance of substance abuse and our weight."

Dr Shahrad Taheri of the University of Bristol presenting research from his obesity clinic to the Department of Health.

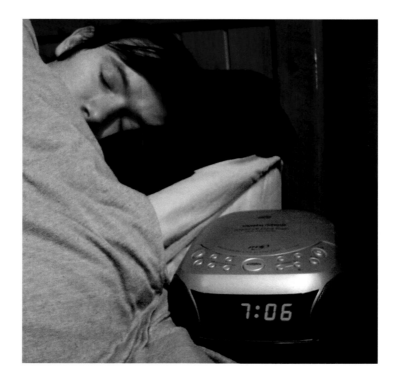

Look after your mental health

Depression

Depression is a huge and very common problem. It affects everyone at some time in their lives. In the UK, about 15% are thought to be clinically depressed. About 4 million people receive antidepressants.

Suicide causes 3,000 deaths a year. Treatment for depression is estimated to cost the NHS £2 billion a year.

Sometimes it is a normal reaction to unhappy circumstances such as a close relative's death or illness, marital problems, stress at work or financial problems. Sometimes it occurs for no good reason, and lifestyle and nutrition may be playing an important part in the cause.

DEPRESSION AND MENTAL HEALTH

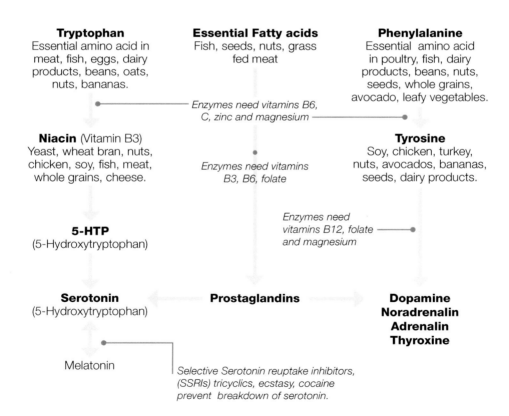

Tryptophan
Essential amino acid in meat, fish, eggs, dairy products, beans, oats, nuts, bananas.

Essential Fatty acids
Fish, seeds, nuts, grass fed meat

Phenylalanine
Essential amino acid in poultry, fish, dairy products, beans, nuts, seeds, whole grains, avocado, leafy vegetables.

Enzymes need vitamins B6, C, zinc and magnesium

Niacin (Vitamin B3)
Yeast, wheat bran, nuts, chicken, soy, fish, meat, whole grains, cheese.

Enzymes need vitamins B3, B6, folate

Tyrosine
Soy, chicken, turkey, nuts, avocados, bananas, seeds, dairy products.

5-HTP
(5-Hydroxytryptophan)

Enzymes need vitamins B12, folate and magnesium

Serotonin
(5-Hydroxytryptophan)

Prostaglandins

Dopamine
Noradrenalin
Adrenalin
Thyroxine

Melatonin

Selective Serotonin reuptake inhibitors, (SSRIs) tricyclics, ecstasy, cocaine prevent breakdown of serotonin.

Anti-depressant medication may be required, but there are other more natural ways to help, which may mean medication can be avoided or given at lower doses with less risk of side effects.

Antidepressants work by slowing the breakdown of serotonin and other neurotransmitters. The boosting of the foods which help to produce important neurotransmitters such as serotonin, noradrenalin, adrenalin, dopamine and acetylcholine seems sensible and can be as effective as medication.

The diagram shows the importance of supplying the essential amino acids to make neurotransmitters but also the necessity of providing essential fatty acids, vitamins and minerals.

Causes of Depression

- Serotonin deficiency causes low mood and insomnia.
- Adrenalin/noradrenalin deficiency causes low motivation.

Low serotonin is caused by:

- Lack of amino acid tryptophan which is a pre-curser to serotonin.(rich in fish, meat, dairy products, soya, beans, oats and eggs). It is also present in smaller amounts in many fruit and vegetables.
- Lack of carbohydrate which stimulates insulin to carry tryptophan into the brain.
- Low sex hormones (oestrogen in women and testosterone in men). Sex hormones block the breakdown of serotonin (like SSRIs)..
- Lack of sunshine and light which stimulates serotonin and sex hormone production.
- Lack of essential fatty acids (needed for serotonin production).
- Lack of co enzyme vitamins and minerals. Including vitamins B3, B6, C. folic acid, magnesium, chromium and zinc. (B6 is an essential co-factor in the synthesis of serotonin).

Other causes:

- Trans-fats - block the conversion of essential fats into vital brain fats such as DHA,GLA and prostaglandins.
- Cigarette smoke - contains many oxidants. It also contains cadmium which accumulates and depletes zinc.
- Excess alcohol - impairs mental performance and acts as a depressant.

Factors other than nutrition that help reduce depression

- Stress reduction: stress such as that from overworking, unemployment, financial or relationship problems and bereavement may cause depression. This may be aggravated by poor nutrition.
- Exercise: study showed that a daily 30 minute walk or jog three times a week is as effective as an antidepressant.
- Light: light has a direct effect on the pineal gland which produces melatonin, an antidepressant. Sunshine stimulates serotonin and sex hormone production. Increasing exposure to natural sunlight helps. For indoor lighting, full spectrum light bulbs may help..
- Negative ions: have an antidepressant effect. Air near waterfalls, mountains, beaches and forests have more negative ions. An Ioniser may be helpful.
- Music: can elevate your mood and reduce stress.
- Meditation: may help reduce stress and depression.
- Socialising and laughter elevate the mood.
- Counsellor or psychotherapist may help. Cognitive therapy has proved more effective than antidepressants in some studies but is not widely available.
- Internet websites such as BluePages and MoodGym may help.
- Advice from a GP, psychiatrist, dietician or nutritionist may help.
- Anti-depressant medication may help.

Depression and Nutrition

A number of studies have shown a correlation between low intakes of fish in a country and a high level of depression among its people. A 1998 Lancet article noted that the more fish the population of a country eats, the lower their incidence of depression. Fish are a good source of Omega-3. Omega-3 supplements have been shown to significantly improve depression and give better results than anti-depressant drugs.

Low levels of certain vitamins and minerals have been noted in depression and bi-polar affective disorder. In studies where supplements have been given there has been as much as a 50% improvement in symptoms. Combining tryptophan or 5HTP supplements with selective serotonin inhibitors (SSRIs) has been found to give better results than SSRIs alone.

A study in 2003 found that high homocysteine levels double the risk of depression. Homocysteine levels can be decreased by reducing meat and dairy product intake and having adequate Vitamin B12, B2, B6, folic acid and zinc.

Depression and sugar

Excess of refined carbohydrates as in white bread, pasta, rice, pastry, biscuits, cakes and most processed foods are associated with depression. Uneven blood sugar with sudden high levels and then low levels causes mood swings with an increased risk of irritability, anxiety, aggressive behaviour, insomnia, fatigue and depression. Refined sugar has very small amounts of nutrients.

The lack of mood-enhancing vitamin B reduces the ability to turn the sugar into energy. The lack of chromium reduces the ability of insulin to control blood sugar levels. Chromium and vitamin B supplements help reduce depression. The lack of magnesium and zinc in refined carbohydrates also contributes to depression.

Cholesterol and Depression

There has been concern that over-enthusiastic lowering of fat and cholesterol may affect mood and increase the risk of depression. This may be related to a decreased production of sex hormones which are made from cholesterol.

- Ten male and ten female volunteers between 20 and 37 year were given a diet containing 41% energy as fat for one month. Then half went onto a low fat diet providing 25% energy from fat. Changes in mood and blood lipids were noted. The low fat diet had an adverse effect on mood with an increase in anxiety, anger and hostility ratings. In the low fat diet group HDL cholesterol was decreased. There was very little change in total cholesterol, LDL cholesterol or triglycerides.

Wells. University of Sheffield 1998

- Men with a low cholesterol level (Less than 4.5 mmol/L) have a higher prevalence of depressive symptoms than those with a cholesterol level between 6 and 7 mmol/L. No difference in anger, hostility and impulsivity were observed.

Steegmans, Dept. Epidemiology. Rotterdam.2000

Important nutrients to avoid depression and anxiety

Tryptophan	Lean meat, dairy, nuts, seeds, beans, vegetables, whole grains, fruit.
Tyrosine	Lean meat, dairy, vegetables, fruit.
GABA	Whole grains.
Vitamin B3	Whole grains, vegetables, nuts, meat, fish, seeds.
Vitamin B6	Whole grains, fruit, fish, vegetables, meat, beans.
Vitamin C	Vegetables, fruit.
Folic acid	Green leafy vegetables, fish, meat, nuts, seeds, beans, fruit.
Chromium	Whole grains, cheese, eggs, meat, brewers yeast.
Magnesium	Green vegetables, nuts, seeds, whole grains, dairy, beans, fruit,
Selenium	Whole grains, meat, fish, seafood, vegetables, nuts, dairy, seeds.
Zinc	Seafood, fish, cereals, nuts, dairy, beans, meat, seeds, vegetables, fruit.
Omega -3	Fish, seeds, nuts, green vegetables.

Important nutrients to avoid Insomnia

Magnesium	Green vegetables, nuts, seeds, dairy, whole grains, fruit.

Important nutrients to help memory and concentration

Vitamin B1	Whole grains, vegetables, seeds, nuts, fish, meat, beans.
Vitamin B5	Whole grains, dairy, fruits, vegetables, beans.
Vitamin B6	Whole grains, fruit, vegetables, meat, beans.
Vitamin B12	Meat, fish, seafood, dairy,
Vitamin E	Whole grains, fish, seeds, nuts, beans.
Omega- 3	Fish, flax seeds, walnuts, green vegetables.
Zinc	Seafood, cereals, nuts, dairy, beans, seeds, veg, fruit.
Selenium	Nuts, seeds, mushrooms, fish.
Coenzyme Q	Oily fish, nuts, seeds, soya.
Glutathione	Garlic, onions, nuts, seeds.

How to reduce anxiety.

- Eat slow releasing carbohydrates rather than high sugar foods or drinks to avoid large fluctuations in blood sugar levels.
- Avoid excess of stimulants such as caffeine and nicotine which increase stress.
- GABA (gamma-amino-butyric acid) is the main calming transmitter. It reduces the effect of excess adrenaline, noradrenalin and dopamine. It makes people relaxed and happy while a deficiency causes anxiety, depression and insomnia. Precursor of GABA is an amino acid taurine. Taurine is highly concentrated in animal foods such as fish, eggs and meat. It is present in the drink Red Bull but unfortunately along with an excess of caffeine and sugar. Vegetarians are more likely to have a deficiency. The synthesis of GABA requires zinc (whole grains, fish, nuts, seeds, fruit, vegetables meat.) The effect of GABA is increased by sleeping tablets and tranquillizers and decreased by stimulants such as caffeine.
- Herbs that reduce anxiety include valerian, kava, hops and passion flower.
- Magnesium helps your mind and muscles relax. Deficiency causes muscle cramps, anxiety and insomnia. Magnesium is in seeds, nuts, fruit and vegetables especially dark green leafy vegetables such as spinach.
- High blood levels of copper increases noradrenalin and anxiety. Modern water pipes are made of copper. Levels of copper are reduced by vitamin C, B3(niacin), folic acid, B12, zinc and manganese.

Addiction

The brain requires sufficient complex carbohydrates, amino acids, essential fatty acids, vitamins, minerals and water to produce neurotransmitters . A good balance of neurotransmitters is essential for good mental health, as they influence mood, memory and concentration.

Some substances have a strong stimulant effect on certain brain transmitters which produce a temporary improvement in mood. Examples are:
Caffeine in tea, coffee, cola and chocolate.

Nicotine in cigarettes

Alcohol

Drugs- cannabis, amphetamines, cocaine, heroin.

When the brain is 'flooded' by an influx of stimulant, the brain receptors respond by "closing down" until the excess is metabolised away. This creates a craving for further stimulant, but, with continued excess stimulation, the neurotransmitter response becomes less sensitive and an increased uptake is required to release the neurotransmitter that the brain is lacking.

Addiction is more likely if there is a deficiency of neurotransmitters such as serotonin, dopamine and noradrenalin and the person feels the need to increase the low levels because of a low mood and feeling of stress and fatigue.

Higher natural levels are provided by sufficient essential amino acids such as tryptophan and phenylalanine, essential fatty acids especially omega 3, vitamins such as B3 (niacin) and minerals such as zinc.

Anti-social behaviour

A fairer society, which would give more reward to the lower paid and less to the overpaid, would help to reduce anti-social behaviour and crime. Adequate housing, reasonable living and working conditions and financial security are important factors.

Poor nutrition, excessive stress and toxins are also important factors in causing poor mental health and making crime and violence more likely. In a number of studies, nutritional supplements given to prisoners and school children have been shown to reduce aggressive and antisocial behaviour. Supplements of Omega-3 and vitamin B have proved helpful. Minerals magnesium, chromium and zinc may help. Also reducing meat, saturated fat, sugar, additives and trans-fats in processed food is beneficial. In general, a more vegetarian diet with more nuts, seeds and fish is recommended.

Neurotoxins and anti-social behaviour

Neurotoxins, such as heavy metals and food additives, may cause reduced intellectual performance and antisocial behaviour.

Lead in exhaust fumes and paint was a cause of aggression and hyperactivity, but this has been reduced by unleaded petrol and lead free paints. Lead level in soil has risen by over 500 times since prehistoric ages. Children with high blood lead levels are found to have reduced mental and physical skills. In 1980's, before the introduction of lead free petrol, it was estimated that lead was damaging the minds of one in two children in Europe.

Cadmium in cigarette smoke may cause aggression and confusion.

Aluminium in tap water and from cookware may cause memory loss and confusion.

Copper from tap water may cause anxiety and paranoia

Mercury in pesticides and large fish may cause memory loss and headaches. The expression 'mad as a hatter' came about in the 19th century when hatters polished top hats with mercury. Mercury is very toxic and small amounts can disturb brain function. Mercury is used in a number of chemical processes. Dumping of industrial waste at sea has increased mercury levels in fish in some areas. Large fish such as shark, marlin, swordfish, salmon and tuna are most affected as they eat smaller fish all containing mercury which accumulates. The toxic effect is decreased by the fact that fish have high selenium levels. Mercury is also present in some tooth fillings and as a constituent of thiomerosal which was formerly used as a preservative in some vaccines. However there has been no evidence that tooth fillings or vaccines have caused adverse effects.

Tartrazine in food colouring may cause hyperactivity and poor concentration. Monosodium glutamate in food additives may cause anxiety and panic attacks.

Detox

Heavy metal poisoning is aggravated by lack of Zinc which is an antagonist of heavy metals. Calcium, vitamin C, magnesium and selenium are also helpful in counteracting the effects of metal toxicity. Certain foods help to detoxify heavy metals. Amino acids methionine and cystine found in garlic, onions and eggs, alginic acid in seaweed, pectin in apples, carrots and citrus fruits all help to chelate and remove heavy metals.

The liver and kidneys are highly efficient at removing toxins from the bloodstream and are not helped by the various pills, juices, teas and oils that are sold for their detoxifying effects. Drinking plenty of water and eating fruit, vegetables and nuts is just as effective.

Manic-Depression

Various degrees of manic depression or bi-polar disorder are very common.

Mood swings may be triggered by blood sugar imbalance. High blood sugar elevates mood and low blood sugar depresses. Manic behaviour may be caused by too much sugar or stimulants such as caffeine, nicotine, drugs and stress.

Food allergy may trigger mania. e.g. wheat allergy.

A deficiency of zinc or lithium may cause mania or depression.

Depressed patients often have low hair lithium levels and may benefit from supplements. Lithium is essential for goats and pigs and may be an essential trace mineral for humans. There is a very low level of lithium in British water supplies. Hair lithium levels were low in 20% of a sample population (2,648) in the U.S. Low lithium levels have been found in people with heart disease, learning difficulties and violent criminal tendencies. Lithium is found in kelp (seaweed) fish and seafood. Excess lithium may dampen emotional expression.

Omega-3 in fish oils is very helpful in manic depression.

Magnesium is a mood stabiliser. Most people are deficient. It is present in vegetables, fruit, nuts and seeds. Zinc, vanadium, vitamin B6, B3 and C are also important.

A mild degree of manic depression occurs in most people and is quite normal. It is only very extreme cases that require treatment. Some people are forced to be manic in order to cope with a very demanding job and may then become depressed if they reach a burnout situation. Creative enthusiasts are prone to overwork themselves and then even if successful have a rebound episode of depression.

Schizophrenia

Schizophrenia has many forms and varies in severity. It is a common problem and diagnosed in about one in a hundred people. Like depression and other mental illnesses, it is possible for anyone to develop symptoms at sometime in their lives, especially if they have a combination of poor nutrition and excessive stress. The illness often occurs in early adult life and is often triggered by a stressful event such as the break-up of a relationship, bereavement, traumatic road accident, excessive workload or intimidation and bullying from workmates or employers. Some people who have a lack of certain enzymes due to their genetic makeup are more susceptible.

One type of schizophrenia is associated with high copper and iron levels together with low zinc and manganese levels.

Symptoms

- Depression
- Phobias
- Anxiety
- Paranoia, unreasonable fears.
- Thought disorders ,delusions
- Hallucinations (auditory or visual)
- Unreasonable or anti-social behaviour.

In the competitive and stressful world of business, professions, politics and religion, it is not surprising that some people develop some, if not all, of these symptoms especially if their nutrition is poor.

A lack of the amino acid tryptophan which is converted to niacin causes pellagra. Pellagra causes the '3 Ds' - dermatitis, diarrhoea and dementia. Other symptoms are headaches, sleep disturbance, thought disorder, anxiety, hallucinations and depression. These are similar to the symptoms of schizophrenia. There were 25,000 cases of pellagra annually in the southern states of the U.S.A. in the early 1900's where corn, lacking in tryptophan and niacin, was the staple food. Pellagra caused a dermatitis with red skin, paranoia and delusions and people with the problem were often referred to as 'red necks'. It took over twenty years to establish the cause, which at first was thought to be an infection. The disease was cured by niacin supplements and this is now added to bread by law.

An absolute deficiency of niacin (vitamin B3 or nicotinic acid) is now rare but may occur in severe malnutrition. It is a good example of how lack of an important nutrient can cause severe mental disease.

Niacin content is high in yeast, wheat bran, nuts, liver, chicken, soya flour, avocados, lean meat and fatty fish. It is low in cheese, milk and eggs but these are rich in the precursor tryptophan.

Acute schizophrenia is helped by niacin supplements but high doses often give intolerable flushing and skin irritation. The best results are obtained by combining niacin supplements with folic acid and B12. Psychiatrist Dr Abram Hoffer in Canada has been using high doses of niacin and vitamin C to treat Schizophrenia successfully for over 40 years. He claims a 90% cure rate on follow up of 5000 patients diagnosed as having schizophrenia.

Lack of niacin reduces the production of the anti-depressant serotonin, but also increases breakdown of noradrenaline and adrenaline to adenochrome, which can cause thought disorder and hallucinations similar to those seen in pellagra and schizophrenia. Some people may have inherited a lack of certain enzymes which makes them more at risk if nutritional deficiencies occur.

Some schizophrenics have food intolerances and improve on a wheat or dairy free diet.

Although it is worth advising a good diet and giving supplements it is doubtful if it will cure all schizophrenics, especially when the disorder has been established for a long time. In these cases, antipsychotic medication may be required, but, even in these cases, nutritional supplements are helpful by enabling a reduced dose of medication with a reduced risk of side effects.

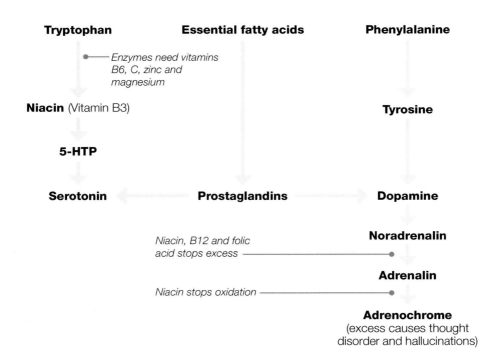

Parkinson's disease

Parkinson's disease is due to a deficiency of dopamine. The cause is not fully understood. A possible factor is that, just as over-stimulation of insulin causes diabetes, over-stimulation of dopamine by stress and stimulants such as caffeine and nicotine, together with inadequate vitamins and minerals to produce dopamine, may cause Parkinson's disease or contribute to the cause. Medication may be required but good nutrition or supplements may help.

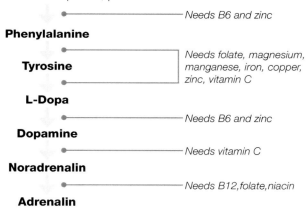

Dietary Protein
containing essential amino acids,
obtained from eggs, fish, meat,
milk, cheese, pulses, soya, cereals,
vegetables such as spinach, peas.

Needs B6 and zinc

Phenylalanine

Needs folate, magnesium, manganese, iron, copper, zinc, vitamin C

Tyrosine

L-Dopa

Needs B6 and zinc

Dopamine

Needs vitamin C

Noradrenalin

Needs B12, folate, niacin

Adrenalin

Poor memory and Dementia

Phospholipids, choline and serine, promote neurotransmission in the brain and help make up the myelin that sheaths all nerves. They improve mood, mental performance and memory.

Acetylcholine, the memory transmitter, is made directly from choline, a phospholipid. A deficiency in it is the most common cause for declining memory. People with Alzheimer's dementia have a marked deficiency of acetylcholine, and the drugs given for dementia mainly work by reducing the breakdown of acetylcholine. The body can make phospholipids and it is therefore not classed as an essential nutrient. However a deficiency may occur especially in the elderly and be helped by a better diet or supplements.

The richest sources of phospholipids in the average diet are egg yolks and organ meats such as liver and kidney. Less of both are eaten today than in the past. Soya beans, wheat germ, peanuts and other nuts are also good sources. Fish especially sardines are rich in choline.

Lecithin is the best source of phospholipids and is present in eggs.

Anticholinergic drugs such as amitriptyline or codeine reduce acetylcholine and may temporarily reduce memory.

Vitamin B1, B5, B12 and vitamin C are essential for the formation of acetylcholine in the body.

Amino acid pyroglutamate increases acetylcholine production and increases the number of acetylcholine receptors. Pyroglutamate is found in fish, dairy products, fruit and vegetables.

Vitamin B3 (Niacin) other B vitamins and zinc are important memory enhancers. Vitamin B and zinc are in whole grains, seeds, nuts, beans, meat and fish.

Vitamin B6(pyridoxine) is essential for GABA synthesis. (Lack of vitamin B6 can cause convulsions in infants and make febrile convulsions more likely). Vitamin B6 is in whole grains, nuts, bananas, fish, meat, vegetables and eggs.

Amino acid glutamine is a precursor of GABA which has a calming influence on the brain and nervous system. Glutamine is the main amino acid in the fluid surrounding the brain and enhances memory and mood. It also reduces addictive tendencies. Glutamine is usually supplied by protein in food but can be synthesised by the body. It is present in meat, fish, beans, eggs and dairy products.

Dementia has become more common over the last 50 years. This is thought to be due to a combination of an aging population, genetic factors, dietary changes and environmental factors.

Most cases of dementia are related to multiple strokes caused by hypertension, cardiac arrhythmias and atherosclerosis. The risk of dementia is decreased by reducing the risk of these problems by sensible nutrition and lifestyle.

Studies of fat intake in many countries suggest that the incidence of dementia is higher in those populations that have:

- A high saturated fat intake.
- A low intake of polyunsaturated fatty acids especially omega-3.
- A low intake of fish.
- A low fruit and vegetable consumption.
- A low intake of vitamins B, C and E.

Dementia is also associated with high homocysteine levels, often caused by low folic acid and vitamin B12 levels. These vitamins help to turn homocysteine into glutathione, an antioxidant and the amino acid SAMe. SAMe is vital for the manufacture of acetylcholine.

How to avoid dementia

- Avoid cardiovascular disease, hypertension, obesity, diabetes, smoking, excess alcohol, stress and toxins.
- Have adequate mental and physical exercise.
- Avoid a high intake of saturated fat (meat and dairy products)
- Avoid trans-fats.(some margarine's and processed foods)
- Have adequate essential fatty acids avoiding an excess of omega-6 compared with omega-3 (oily fish, seeds, nuts, green vegetables).
- Have adequate protein to supply the essential amino acids choline, glutamine and other precursors of acetylcholine (fish, eggs, fruit and vegetables.)
- Have adequate folic acid (green leafy veg, carrots, whole grains, eggs, avocados, melon) and B12 (liver, meat, eggs, milk, cheese and seaweed) to keep homocysteine levels down.
- Have adequate vitamins especially Vitamins A, B, C and E (fruit, vegetables, nuts, wholegrain cereals and bread.)
- Have adequate minerals especially zinc, chromium and magnesium, (wholemeal cereal and bread, nuts, seeds, beans, fish and meat).

Avoid over and under-working

Work brings self esteem, companionship and money. Unemployment brings loss of self esteem, social isolation and poverty. Unemployed people are more likely to have a smoking, alcohol or drug addiction, medical and psychiatric problems. They are more likely to be involved in crime. They attend GP's and hospitals frequently. A depressive episode is common, and may have been caused by excess stress from the previous work or marital problems. The boredom and stress of unemployment then prolongs the depression. Increasing employment brings great health and financial benefits to the individual and to a society.

People in the UK, on average, work harder and longer than any in Europe.

Overworking and excessive prolonged stress can lead to a burnout situation with severe depression. ('All work and no play make Jack a dull boy'). Life is becoming increasingly complex and hectic partly because of better technology and communication such as from mobile phones and e-mails. Financial debt and financial anxiety are more common. People are more mobile and have less family support. There is less religious belief and support. Marital breakdown and divorce is more common. The average diet is poor. People in the UK are among the highest alcohol and drug consumers. Depression rates in urban UK (17%) are higher than the rest of Europe and Scandinavia. (Spain 2.6% ,Finland 5.9%).

Overworking

Stress causes the release of the hormone cortisone and adrenaline which prepares us for 'fight or flight'. This would have been associated with encountering wild animals in the past, but is now associated with threats to our social status and financial future.

A certain amount of stress is beneficial and stimulating. However, continuous high levels of stress and raised cortisone levels eventually cause a fall in serotonin, dopamine and noradrenalin levels. High cortisol levels are linked to increased activity in the right frontal brain. This causes fearfulness, irritability and withdrawal from others. It also reduces the effectiveness of our immune system and aggravates osteoporosis. Lowered serotonin causes lowered mood, increased impulsiveness, aggression, reduced concentration and memory. The depleted dopamine causes reduced motivation and the suppression of the pleasure neurotransmitters, endorphin and encephalin, which are vital for forming strong social bonds.

Burnout

Severe occupational stress or burnout may be linked with job dissatisfaction but is mainly due to a prolonged excessive workload. There are three main components.:

1. Emotional exhaustion:

Tiredness, irritability and depression,

Damage to interpersonal relationships.

Increased risk of marital problems and divorce.

Poor concentration leading to frequent mistakes and accidents.

Increased risk of car accidents.

Increased risk of alcohol and drug abuse.

2. Depersonalisation:

Loss of sense of compassion.

Loss of sense of humour.

3. Lack of personal accomplishment and low productivity .

The constant backlog of work leads to more stress and low self esteem.

Workload

There is an optimum workload which is healthy. It contributes to our mental and physical health and produces happiness. A lack of work or an excessive workload may cause depression.

People more likely to suffer burnout are those:

- With over conscientious, obsessive, inflexible, perfectionist personality traits.
- With high personal moral standards.
- Who are anxious to please and have difficulty in saying "no".
- Who are reluctant to delegate.
- Who fear failing to keep up with colleagues.

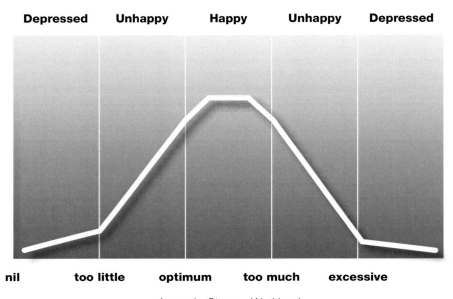

| Depressed | Unhappy | Happy | Unhappy | Depressed |

Performance (vertical axis)

| nil | too little | optimum | too much | excessive |

Arousal - Stress - Workload

Modified from Yerkes-Dodson Law 1908

Long working hours

US researchers studied 34 medical residents after they had worked an 80 to 90 hour week for a month, and after they had worked a 44 hour week for a month and then consumed the alcohol equivalent of four cocktails immediately before being tested. Those who had worked long hours were 30% less likely to maintain a steady speed on a driving simulator than those who had been drinking.

JAMA 2005

A US study looked at 11,000 Americans workers, their job histories, schedules and the occurrence of injury or illness between 1987 and 2000. It was found that jobs with overtime carried a 61% higher hazard rate. Working 12 hour days was associated with a 37% higher hazard rate. Working a 60 hour week was associated with a 23% higher hazard rate. Conclusion: Long working hours generate workplace accidents and mistakes due to tiredness. They also cause more accidents and illness outside work.

Occup Environ Med 2005

Employers and people with social and financial security have less risk of stress symptoms and depression. They need to recognize that people who are less fortunate require a sense of security, support and encouragement rather than constant criticism and bullying. The workforce would be happier and more efficient. There would be a decrease in absenteeism and sickness. We are designed biologically to be part of a social group and feel happier if we are welcomed and supported by the other members of the group. Ideally we should be part of a family group, working group and a hobby group. Some benefit from a religious group. Research shows monkeys kept in solitary confinement rapidly drop their serotonin levels and become depressed.

Personality

To enable a long life it is important to inherit the right personality.

Type A1.Ambitious, hardworking, ruthless and over confident. They have a desire to dominate at home and work. They enjoy danger and taking risks. They tend to work too hard and play too hard. Often accident prone, impulsive, aggressive and impatient. Morals may be suspect (A flexible conscience). Often have more than one wife or husband.

Type A2. May be ambitious and over-conscientious, highly strung, worrying, insomniac workaholics. Not dominating, lack confidence, avoid risk. Sincere, high moral code. Need support of a good wife or husband to whom they stay faithful.

Type B: Often clever, charming, laid back, cope with any situation, seldom angry or aggressive. Avoid competition, May lack motivation and ambition or be lazy. Make good husbands and wives.

A person with type A personality may be the most successful but is more likely to suffer from, stress, anxiety, depression, cardiovascular disease and a shortened life.

Megalomaniacs

We should all discourage rather than encourage megalomaniacs. Our society is remarkably tolerant of, and has an odd tendency to admire, some megalomaniacs.

Extreme megalomaniac examples are :

The Pharaohs who built the Pyramids as tombs.

The Chinese emperor who created the terracotta soldiers.

Rulers who build multiple palaces and monuments to themselves.

The Creators of excessively large Country houses and Chateaux.

In all these extreme cases, poor people were made to work excessively hard for very little reward in order to create something which has very little use except for the glorification of the creator.

The Boss

Who you work for can make a big difference to your stress levels and mental health. Ambitious workaholics, who often have to strive for unreasonable targets, are common at the top of business, politics, professions and all walks of life. It has become almost essential to be a workaholic to compete in the excessive and unnecessary pace of modern society. In its mildest form, these people can be of great help to a society. They work hard, take responsibility and create wealth and jobs. Some are considerate and look after those less fortunate. Some cause considerable stress, anxiety and depression in those people working for them and living with them. Some strive for an unwarranted and unnecessarily high income and an excess of material possessions. Some have a large number of homes, cars, boats and planes but are still unhappy and strive for more.

The Big M syndrome

If possible avoid working for someone with the 'Big M syndrome'. This is the Money grubbing, Masochistic, Megalomaniac. These people can be very successful as they are often ruthless about getting to a position of wealth and power. They are often workaholics who are willing to punish themselves in order to achieve a goal. They may despise others who do not do the same and become sadistic bullies. They can be extremely inconsiderate, selfish and demanding. Social and financial power reduces their risk of stress and depression, but they do not feel guilty about inducing it in others. To extend their power or wealth, they are willing to go to war with other people or nations often using fundamental religion or politics as an excuse. They like to control people and can drive some of their most able supporters to a burnout situation. If the able person tries to escape from control they can be unmercifully victimised. The 'Big M' syndrome can be recognised in all walks of life.

Do not take religion and politics too seriously

If being enthusiastic about religion or politics helps you to make a contribution towards helping other people, that's fine. However, remember that all the laws and opinions in religion, politics and the law are made by other men and not by some higher intelligence. ("The golden rule is that there is no golden rule" (Bernard Shaw)). Intelligent men and women are usually well read, but, even if well intentioned, can sometimes be misinformed, obsessive, dogmatic and completely wrong. They may also have a vested interest. If it makes you want to bring harm on other people who do not think in the same way as you, religion and politics can be bad for your health as well as other peoples.

Respect for authority, including scientific, political and religious leaders, is important . However, their limitations should be recognized.

"The greatest enemy of knowledge is not ignorance, it is the illusion of knowledge."

Stephen Hawking

"An expert is a man who has stopped thinking – he knows!"

Frank Lloyd Wright

"Ignorance more frequently begets confidence than does knowledge; it is those who know little, and not those who know much, who so positively assert that this or that problem will never be solved by science."

Charles Darwin.

Postscript

We can learn from history.

In the 16th, 17th and 18th century there were many voyages to discover and claim new lands. Scurvy began to affect the sailors after about six weeks at sea and caused loose teeth, bleeding gums and haemorrhages. Many of the sailors on these long voyages suffered or died from scurvy. For example, in 1619, Jens Munk commanded a Danish discovery expedition to Hudson Bay, Canada. Struck down by scurvy at Churchill River, out of a crew of 64, only Munk and two others survived to sail their ship home.

In the early days of long voyages sailors were aware of scurvy and were given fruit such as oranges and lemons to prevent it. The Chinese navies grew fruit and vegetables in huge pots on their ships. The British Navy issued lemon juice rations diluted with water. The Dutch developed large lemon orchards and were by far the largest supplier. They sold the lemons at enormous prices. Because the price of lemons rose in about 1740, the Navy cut the ration of lemon juice to one third. With an inadequate amount of vitamin C, scurvy returned as a major problem for the next fifty years.

As the sailors were getting some lemon juice, the doctors concluded that scurvy was not a deficiency disease and was caused by abnormal humoural factors. Adhering to the then fashionable and so called 'ancient wisdom' and humoural theory, the doctors at that time believed that the basic four humours, blood, phlegm, yellow bile and black bile, were out of balance. To treat scurvy using the humoural hypothesis, the doctors depended on toxic drugs and the value of food was forgotten.

At this time a Dutch doctor Johan Bachstrom wrote about scurvy. "This evil is solely owing to a total abstinence from fresh vegetable food and greens which is alone the true primary cause of the disease". He condemned the use of mercury, alum, nitre, oil of vitriol and other mineral and fossil remedies. Because of his views, he was dismissed and then imprisoned where he died aged 56 years.

In 1747, James Lind, a Scottish naval surgeon serving on HMS Salisbury, carried out experiments on scurvy. He noted that "the number of seamen in time of war who died of shipwreck, capture, famine, fire or sword are but inconsiderable in respect of such as are destroyed by the ship diseases, and by the usual maladies of intemperate climates". Lind could have dismissed the disease as due to infection or 'humours' but luckily for the sailors he considered a nutritional deficiency and carried out a trial.

Lind selected twelve men from the ship who were suffering from scurvy. He split them into six pairs, and gave each pair different additions to their basic diet.

Two received a quart of cider a day,

Two received an unspecified elixir,

Two were given seawater,

Two received garlic, mustard and horseradish,

Two received vinegar

Two were given two oranges and one lemon every day.

Four groups reported no change. Those on cider showed a slight improvement. Those on oranges and lemon experienced a remarkable recovery. Lind had definitively established the superiority of citrus fruits above all other remedies.

I am sure today the trial would have been deemed as not being large enough to show statistical evidence and the results not published. It does demonstrate, though, how any doctor who can observe a disease or problem and consider all possibilities (including enviromental factors and nutrition) can carry out a useful mini trial.

Lind published a treatise of the scurvy in 1754, but it was not until more than 40 years later that an official Admiralty order was issued on the supply of lemon juice to ships. Almost immediately after this order, scurvy disappeared from the fleets and naval hospitals, and the annual number of sick sailors sent to the hospitals was halved. Captain James Cook's sailors in his three year voyage of discovery around the world in 1768 benefited from the recognition that lack of fresh fruit caused illness and drank lemon and lime juice. By 1800 the royal navy was again issuing limes and lemons. This is thought to have helped the defeat of Napoleon whose navy was not so well informed. The British sailors were given the nickname 'The Limeys'.

The nutrient in citrus fruit responsible for curing scurvy was not recognised as Vitamin C until 1912.It was synthesised in 1935.

This is a good example of how the evidence on the cause of a disease changed over time and why doctors must keep an open mind when considering various therapies.

In particular it shows that prevention of disease is the ideal. Doctors are well placed to give advice about lifestyle and nutrition which can prevent disease. Many already do this but some lack an in depth knowledge of nutritional factors as it is not given a high enough priority in their education.

Most doctors are keen to practice evidence based medicine and help their patients as much as possible, but they can be influenced by the marketing skills of those with a vested interest in promoting certain fashions and products. Today there is much more scrutiny and true evidence than in the days of the 'humoral' theory and 'blood-letting' but we must still be on our guard.

The Polypill

In 2003 the Polypill was announced with great publicity in the British Medical Journal (BMJ) This was a pill to prevent 80% of heart attacks and is still being considered for mass medication of people in the future.

The polypill consisted of six constituents, all of which were known to reduce the risk of coronary heart disease (CHD) and stroke. The risk factors that would be reduced were blood pressure, cholesterol, hypertension, homocysteine and platelet stickiness.

The constituents were:

Statin: Atorvastatin 10 mg reduces LDL cholesterol and CHD by...... 46%

Thiazide.

Angiotensin 2 receptor antagonist.

Calcium channel blocker:
All at half standard dose reduce blood pressure and CHD by 46%

Folic acid: 0.8mg daily reduces homocysteine and CHD by 24%

Aspirin: 75mg daily reduces platelet stickiness and CHD by 16%

Combined effect on reducing CHD 88%
and reducing stroke 80%

If given from age 55, about one third of the people would benefit.

On average each would gain 11-12 years of life free from a heart attack or stroke. Adverse effects from the medication would occur in 8-15% of people.

(BMJ. June 28 2003)

Research by Department of Environmental Medicine.
Barts, London and Queen Marys Hospitals. London.
Prof. Wald and Prof. Law.
Examination of 354 randomised controlled trials.

The Polymeal

A year later the Polymeal was announced in the BMJ. There was very little publicity. It was offered as a more natural, safer and tastier alternative to the Polypill. It would also be a lot less expensive. The Polymeal also contained six constituents which were known to reduce the risk of coronary heart disease and stroke.

Wine: 150 ml of wine daily reduces CHD by 32%

Fish: 114g consumed four times a week reduces CHD by 14%

Dark Chocolate: 100g daily reduces BP and CHD by 21%

Fruit and Vegetables: 400g daily reduces BP and CHD by 21%

Garlic: 2.7g daily reduces cholesterol and CHD by 25%

Almonds: 68g daily reduces cholesterol and CHD by 12.5%

Combined effect on reduction of CHD events for men was 76%
Increase in total life expectancy of 6.6 years, (4.8 in women)
Increase of life expectancy free from CHD of 9 years, (8.1 in women).

The authors noted that these foods had been enjoyed by humankind for many centuries and that finding happiness in a frugal, active lifestyle could spare us a future of pills and hypochondria.

(BMJ Dec.18 2004)

Research by Department of public health, Holland.
Belgian Health care Knowledge centre.
Department of Epidemiology and Preventive Medicine. Australia.
Drs. Franco, Bonneux, de Laet, Peeters, Steyerberg and Mackenbach.

Data from Framingham heart study and many other references.

Beware of Statistics

The use of relative risk rather than absolute risk in statistics does exaggerate the value of both drugs and foods. For example if 1% of people on a drug had a heart attack while 2% on placebo had a heart attack the reduced absolute risk is 1% but the reduced relative risk is 50%. Doctor's, newspaper editors and the public are much more likely to be impressed by a drug which reduces a disease by 50% rather than the more accurate figure of 1%.

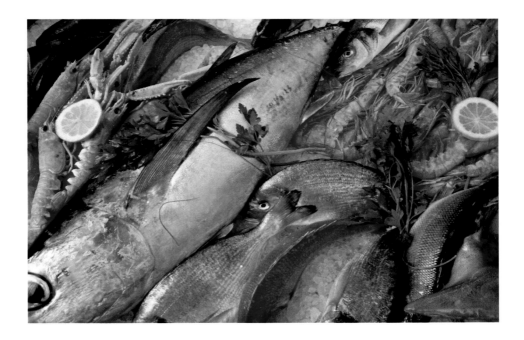

Summary advice

How to avoid coronary heart disease.

Avoid being overweight: If BMI over 25 risk: increases times three.

Avoid smoking: Over 20 cigarettes a day risk: increases times three.

Avoid trans fats in processed foods: risk increases times two.

Avoid saturated fats in animal products: They raise cholesterol.

Avoid excess refined carbohydrates/sugar. They raise triglycerides.

Avoid excess salt: causes hypertension.

Increase anti-oxidants (e.g. vitamins C, E, Flavonoids).

Increase oily fish and essential vegetable fatty acids: especially omega 3.

Increase B vitamins (B6, B12, Folic acid): Lower homocysteine.

Increase fibre

Have alcohol in moderation, (preferably red wine)

Exercise.

Control cholesterol. Reduce LDL and triglycerides. Raise HDL.

Control blood pressure.

How to avoid or help diabetes.

Avoid obesity by avoiding excess food and having adequate exercise.

Avoid excess **sugar** in food and drinks.

Avoid excess **alcohol** especially beer which contains the high G.I. sugar maltose.

Avoid **processed foods** such as biscuits, cakes, snack bars which tend to be high in refined sugar and trans-fats. They are very low in chromium and cause the body to lose chromium when they raise the blood sugar.

Avoid an excess of fried food and crisps which contain **trans-fats.**

Avoid an excess of **cow's meat and dairy products** to avoid an excess of hormones such as insulin growth factor and steroids .

Have low glycaemic index (G.I.) carbohydrate as in wholegrain bread, pasta, vegetables and fruit. Wholegrain bread and cereals are low G.I. and provide fibre and essential nutrients such as chromium which helps insulin work and reduces insulin resistance. Chromium is also in meat, cheese and egg yolk. Fruit and vegetables have very little chromium and refined grain products such as white bread almost none. Smoking and excess caffeine can also deplete chromium.

Have oat bran which contains beta-glucan a nutrient which has a marked effect on reducing blood sugar and also LDL cholesterol. It is low G.I. and also provides fibre. Oat bran is present with oak flakes in cereals, porridge and oat cakes.

How to avoid high blood pressure

Reduce sodium intake by reducing Salt

Reduce Homocysteine levels by: reducing meat, cheese and other proteins in diet. Increase vitamins B2, B6, B12, Folic acid and Zinc to help metabolize homocysteine.

Avoid excess saturated fat in meat and dairy products.

Avoid excess of coffee and tea which increase homocysteine levels.

Avoid excess alcohol.

Avoid excess weight.

Avoid smoking.

Avoid stress

Increase magnesium, calcium, potassium and fibre intake by having adequate fruit, vegetables, yeast, brown rice, soybeans, nuts and seeds. Eating just two bananas a day can lower blood pressure by 10%. Fruit and vegetables, contain potassium which helps the body excrete sodium.

Eat a Mediterranean type diet with fresh tomatoes, garlic, oily fish, olive oil and red wine. These all improve the health of the arteries and heart.

Have adequate omega-3 essential fatty acids to reduce blood stickiness and the health of the arterial walls. Peripheral resistance is decreased.

Have adequate exercise.

How to make the blood less sticky and reduce blood pressure

Making the blood less sticky improves the circulation and reduces the risk of thrombosis and high blood pressure. Thrombosis may cause a stroke, heart attack, deep vein leg thrombosis or pulmonary embolus.

Omega-3 foods reduce the clotting time of blood – omega-3 can be obtained from oily fish such as mackerel, herring, sardines, salmon, tuna and trout or from vegetarian sources such as flax, hemp seeds, walnuts and their oils, mustard seeds, pumpkin seeds, leafy green vegetables. Although omega-3 and omega-6 fatty acids are both essential, the balance is important. An excess of omega-6 relative to omega-3 can increase the risk of thrombosis.

Certain **fruit and vegetables**, particularly tomatoes but also strawberries, grapefruit and melons, contain a component, named P3 that reduces platelet activity and the risk of thrombosis.

Garlic reduces blood platelet stickiness as well as reducing cholesterol.

Turmeric a yellow spice in Indian food, reduces platelet stickiness and relaxes arteries.

Ginkgo biloba reduces platelet stickiness.

Vitamins C reduces blood stickiness **and beta-carotene in fruit and vegetables** also help improve the circulation.

Wearing appropriate clothing and warm food and drinks help.

How to avoid Depression_

Nutritional factors

> **Have adequate intake of amino acid tryptophan** (precursor of serotonin) present in fish, beans, and oats, It is also present in eggs, meat and dairy products but an excess of these should be avoided..

> **Have adequate essential fatty acids** avoiding an excess of Omega-6 compared with Omega-3 (more fish, seeds, nuts and grass fed meat less corn and grain fed meat.)

Avoid excess sugar in foods (e.g. biscuits, cakes, Jams)

Have slow acting low GI carbohydrates with fibre.

Avoid very sweet drinks containing sugar.

Have adequate fruit and vegetables to supply sufficient vitamins, minerals and phytochemicals.

Have wholemeal bread and cereals to provide vitamin B, minerals such as chromium and essential fatty acids.

Avoid excess of Alcohol.

Factors other than nutrition

Exercise. Study showed that a daily 30 minute walk or jog three times a week is as effective as an antidepressant.

Light has a direct effect on the pineal gland which produces melatonin and serotonin, an antidepressant.

For indoor lighting, full spectrum light bulbs may help.

Negative ions have an antidepressant effect. Air near waterfalls, mountains, beaches and forests have more negative ions.

Ioniser may be helpful.

Music can elevate your mood.

Socialising and laughter elevate the mood.

A counsellor or psychotherapist may help. Cognitive therapy has proved more effective than antidepressants in some studies but is not widely available. Internet websites such as BluePages and MoodGym may help.

Anti-depressant medication may help

How to avoid dementia

Avoid cardiovascular disease, hypertension, obesity, diabetes, smoking. Excess alcohol, stress and toxins.

Have adequate mental and physical exercise.

Avoid a high intake of saturated fat and protein (meat and dairy products)

Avoid trans-fats (some margarine and processed foods).

Have adequate essential fatty acids avoiding an excess of omega-6 compared with omega-3 (oily fish, seeds. nuts)

Have adequate but not excess protein to supply the essential amino acids choline, glutamine and other precursors of acetylcholine. (fish, eggs, fruit and vegetables).

Have adequate folic acid (green leafy vegetables, carrots, whole grains, eggs avocados, melon) and B12 (liver, meat, eggs, milk, cheese and seaweed) to keep homocysteine levels down.

Have adequate vitamins especially vitamins A, B, C and E. (fruit, vegetables, nuts, wholegrain cereals and bread.)

Have adequate minerals especially zinc. (nuts, seeds, beans, fish and meat).

How to reduce eye problems

Phytochemicals lutein and zeaxanthin, lower the risk of age related macular degeneration (AMD) and cataracts. They are found in the macula and help to protect the eye from UV light damage. Good sources are dark green and yellow fruit and vegetables. e.g. spinach, cabbage, broccoli, peas, sweet corn, tomatoes, oranges and melon. **Anthocyanins** are plant phytochemicals which help to strengthen blood vessels and reduce the risk of haemorrhage. They are found in dark coloured fruit and vegetables such as raspberries, strawberries, red grapes, blackberries and red cabbage.

Essential fatty acids especially omega-3 are essential for the structure and repair of retinal cells. Found in oily fish, walnuts, flax seed, soy and grass fed meat or eggs.

Vitamin A is essential for healthy eyes. It helps to form rhodopsin, a pigment that is important for night vision. It reduces the risk of AMD and cataracts. Vitamin A in the form of retinol is found in milk, butter, cheese, eggs, oily fish and liver and as beta-carotene in yellow, red and orange fruits and vegetables and dark green vegetables, e.g. carrots, tomatoes, apricots, mangos and spinach.

Vitamin C reduces the risk of cataracts and glaucoma. It is present in all fruit and vegetables. Good sources are citrus fruits, peppers, tomatoes and berries.

Vitamin E may reduce the risk of cataract and strengthens the arteries. It is found in vegetable oils, nuts, eggs, wholegrain and green leafy vegetables.

Avoiding a high sugar and high dairy intake helps reduce the risk of cataracts and glaucoma. High blood sugars due to excess refined sugar or galactose (the sugar in milk) can cause a toxic effect in the eyes due to the production of sorbitol. This causes swelling of the lens and eye tissues. If the situation continues the lens becomes gradually damaged and misty. The drainage of fluid at the front of the eye can be reduced leading to high pressure and glaucoma which eventually puts pressure on the retina at the back of the eye and causes reduced vision.

Deficiency of chromium is thought to increase the risk of raised intraocular pressure and glaucoma. This is thought to be due to the fact that chromium helps the eye muscles to contract. Chromium also helps insulin reduce the blood sugar levels and its toxic effect on the eye. Chromium deficiency and eye muscle weakness may be partly responsible for our difficulty in accommodating near and far vision and the high percentage of people in the western world requiring glasses. Chromium is almost completely removed when bread, sugar or rice is refined. It is in wholemeal bread, nuts, prunes, meat and seafood.

How to help asthma

Low **selenium and vitamin E** levels in pregnancy seem to increase the risk of having an asthmatic child but family history is more important, (nuts in particular Brazil nuts are high in selenium. Ten Brazil nuts give enough selenium for a week). Vitamin E is in vegetable oils, whole grains, nuts, fish, meat and leafy green vegetables.

Breast feeding and delaying the introduction of cow's milk protein until after 6 months seems to reduce the possibility or severity of asthma.

Essential fatty acids in particular omega-3 seem to reduce the incidence or severity of asthma by keeping the prostaglandins in balance.

Adequate Vitamins such as **vitamin B and C and minerals such as zinc** help.

Avoid excess of milk products and meat.

Avoid allergens such as house dust mite, pollens and animal fur.

Avoid smoking. Also avoid inhaling other toxins such as exhaust fumes.

Avoid an excess of aerosol sprays (other than those used to treat asthma). e.g. air fresheners, deodorants, hairsprays and insecticides.

Avoid an excess of nitrites. These occur in cured meats such as salami, bacon, hot-dogs, sausages and ham. They produce reactive forms of nitrogen which can have a damaging effect on the lungs.

How to avoid Osteoporosis

Avoid a high protein diet. Protein –rich foods such as meat and fish are acid forming. These foods are essential for bone health as the framework of bones is protein-based, however too much protein increases calcium excretion.

Avoid hydrogenated fats (Trans-fats) present in fast foods and ready meals. Vitamin K is needed for a strong bone structure. Vegetable oils contain vitamin K but the process of hydrogenation that occurs to make them into margarine and hard cooking fats changes vitamin K's structure so that it no longer strengthens bone and it now blocks the absorption of natural vitamin K.

Avoid high sugar or sweet diet – low in nutrients.

Avoid Cola drinks contains phosphoric acid which increases calcium excretion.

Avoid excess vitamin A (over 1500mcg retinol equivalents) in liver, cod liver oil.

Avoid excess Sulphate increases calcium loss (high dose Glucosamine sulphate may do this).

Avoid excess alcohol.

Avoid smoking tobacco.

Avoid salty processed foods. Increases urinary calcium loss.

Avoid excess stress increases cortisol.

Avoid excess coffee.

Factors reducing Osteoporosis

Have adequate:

Calcium: calcium rich foods are meat, milk and cheese but calcium is better obtained from plants such as green vegetables, herbs and grains to avoid a high protein diet.

Vitamin D helps absorb calcium. In fish and vegetable oils and from sunshine.

Protein (but not excess) in meat or vegetables, nuts, seeds, and wholegrain.

Vitamin K stimulates osteoblasts. Present in green vegetables such as spinach, broccoli and cabbage. Also in vegetable oils that are not hydrogenated such as olive oil.

Fruit and vegetables – alkali forming foods and contain essential nutrients such as vitamin C and K, potassium and magnesium.

Magnesium and manganese in beans and spinach.

Silicon in green beans, lentils, cereals, pasta, bread, pizza, coffee and beer.

Zinc, copper, boron, molybdenum and phosphate. Vitamin B6

Isoflavines (plant hormones with a similar structure to human estrogens) seem to increase bone density. Soya beans and lentils are rich in isoflavones.

Essential fatty acids – Omega-3 and -6.

Fluoride. in water and tea.

Carbonated mineral water – rich in bicarbonate and alkaline. This helps to buffer acid in the blood and decrease calcium taken from bones. It contains calcium and silica both important for bone health.

Exercise preferably weight bearing.

Sunshine to enable skin to produce vitamin D. Thirty minutes of modest skin exposure provides daily requirement.

Anti-inflammatory diet

An anti-inflammatory diet reduces depression, anxiety, dementia, asthma, cardiovascular disease, irritable bowel disease, osteoarthritis and cancer.

Adequate intake of 0mega-3 and omega-6 fatty acids.

Omega-3: oily fish, nuts and seeds, grass fed meat or dairy products.

Omega-6: avoid excess of processed omega-6 vegetable oils e.g. corn, cottonseed, safflower vegetable oils.

Correct ratio is thought to be one portion of omega-3 to three portions of omega 6.

Avoid trans-fats

Reduce insulin production by having **low sugar, low GI diet.**

Avoid excess of saturated fat, meat and dairy products.

Have organic (grass fed) meat and poultry eggs if possible but avoid excess.

Have occasional organ meats (offal) and fish eggs but avoid excess.

Avoid smoking, excess stress and excess alcohol.

Increase antioxidants. e.g. Fruit ,vegetables, beans, wholemeal cereals, bread, nuts and seeds.

Have adequate minerals especially zinc, iodine and selenium.

In nuts, seeds, whole grains, fish, eggs, meat and vegetables,

Use rapeseed or olive oil for occasional frying.

Use flax oil or olive oil for salad dressing.

Anti-cancer advice

Antioxidants help prevent and even reverse the cell and DNA damage that precedes cancer as well as other conditions associated with ageing such as coronary heart disease, strokes and dementia.

Fruit and vegetables are a good source of vitamins and minerals that act as anti-oxidants. They also contain numerous anti-cancer phytonutrients. Include a mixture of different coloured plant foods in your diet to get the correct balance of phytonutrients. Good cancer –preventing foods include broccoli, brussels sprouts, spinach, cabbage, red peppers, beetroot, tomatoes, onions, kale, beans, plums, oranges, lemons and all types of berries and nuts. Garlic, green and black tea, liquorice and turmeric.

Phytoestrogens in certain plants have a weak oestrogen effect and bind to the same receptor sites as the much stronger human oestrogen. They help to prevent oestrogen overload and certain cancers such as those of breast and uterus. Phyto-oestrogens are in lentils, nuts, seeds and beans especially soya. The **high fibre** in vegetables reduces the risk of colon cancer by 40%.

Avoid toxins such as tobacco, radiation and heavy metals. Also avoid xeno-oestrogens which attach to oestrogen receptor sites and promote hormonal cancers. They are present in plastics, some detergents and pesticides.

Avoid an excess of meat, dairy products and eggs to reduce hormones. Especially oestrogen and insulin growth factor.

Avoid trans-fats which increase inflammation and the risk of cancer.

Foods that increase energy and libido

A low GI diet with slow and prolonged acting carbohydrates.

Foods that **increase dopamine**.

Tyrosine – meat, shellfish, fish, eggs, milk, beans and nuts.

Vitamin B12 – meat, liver, eggs, milk, beans and nuts.

Folic acid – green vegetables, avocado, fortified cereal.

Magnesium – milk, nuts and seeds.

Iron – meat, fish, beans, apricots, dark green vegetables and nuts.

Zinc – shellfish, wholegrain bread and muesli.

Phytoestrogens can mimic oestrogen and benefit women's libido in Soya bean products, yogurt, lentils, wholemeal bread and chickpeas.

Omega-3 and antioxidants improve circulation.

Omega-3 fatty acids in oily fish, flax seeds and grass fed meat.

Antioxidants in berries, fruit, vegetables and tea.

Factors that improve fertility

It is important to have adequate:

Vitamins A, B (especially B6, B12 and folic acid) , C and E .

Minerals Zinc, iron, selenium and magnesium.

Protein, carbohydrate and fat.

It is important to avoid:

Excess of protein, sugar, saturated fat with hormones, omega-6, trans-fats, vitamin A and additives.

The risk of miscarriage may be reduced by decreasing meat and dairy intake. This reduces oestrogen and other hormones contained in the saturated fat. Relative progesterone deficiency compared to oestrogen seems to be a cause of miscarriage. Reducing protein intake also reduces homocysteine levels. High homocysteine levels are associated with miscarriage. Adequate vitamin B12 and folate help to reduce homocysteine levels.

A deficiency or imbalance of prostaglandins caused by a deficiency or imbalance of omega-3 and omega-6 essential fatty acids may be an important factor. A deficiency of omega-3 may affect development of the foetus. An excess of omega-6 causes an excess of prostaglandin 2 which may stimulate the uterus to contract. To obtain adequate omega-3 have oily fish, wholemeal bread and green leafy vegetables. Have a small amount of meat, milk and eggs from grass fed animals and reduce corn products and processed foods which tend to have more omega-6 than omega-3.

Reduce refined and processed food to avoid trans-fats.

Avoid an excess of additives such as aspartame and monosodium glutamate.

How to have a healthy child

About 5% of children show evidence of a developmental defect at birth.

Any severe nutritional deficiency can cause birth abnormalities. In particular folic acid, B12 and other B vitamins, minerals zinc, iron, calcium and magnesium and iodine deficiencies have been linked with birth abnormalities.

Avoid an excess of vitamins in particular vitamin A which may increase the risk of birth abnormalities, (too much liver, cod liver oil or supplements may cause excess.)

Avoid excess exposure to toxins such as lead, cadmium, copper and mercury. Fish are important to supply essential fatty acids but excess large fish may cause a toxic intake of mercury.

Essential fatty acids such as omega-3 are important. They are present in green vegetables, nuts, beans, fish and grass fed animal meat.

Avoid an excess of meat and dairy products which raise homocysteine levels.

Excess cigarette smoking, alcohol or drugs intake may all increase the risk of birth abnormalities..

A good diet provides 400mcg of folic acid. 800mcg is optimal. A study of 23,000 women found that those who supplemented their diet with 400mcg of folic acid during the first six weeks of pregnancy had a 75% lower incidence of neural tube defect compared with those who did not.

Breast feeding gives optimum nutrition and reduces the risk of infections, eczema, asthma, obesity and diabetes in the child.

How to help your thyroid

The thyroid hormones determine our rate of metabolism. A deficiency slows down metabolism causing a reduction in physical and mental abilities. The thyroid hormones are formed by an amino acid Tyrosine and Iodine.

Tyrosine is obtained from chicken, turkey, nuts, seeds, avocados, soya, bananas and dairy products. Tyrosine can also be made from another amino acid, phenylalanine which is present in similar foods and additionally in green leafy plants, whole grains and fish.

Iodine is present in fish and seaweed. There is very little in fruit and vegetables and this is dependant on the soil content.

Essential fatty acids play an important role in thyroxin production.

Vitamins A, B2, B3, B6, C and E are required for the synthesis of thyroxin.

Minerals **copper, magnesium, manganese, selenium and zinc** are also essential.

Other halogens like chlorine and fluoride compete with iodine.

Excess of chlorine from drinking water and excess of fluoride in some water or tea may reduce thyroid production.

An excess of oestrogen can block conversion of thyroxine (T4) to the more active T3.

Cooking

The major anti-oxidants in meat, eggs and milk are largely destroyed by cooking. The anti-oxidants in fruit and vegetables are more likely to survive cooking and some may become more available but they may be lost with over-cooking.

Minerals such as magnesium and potassium may be lost in boiling water.

Water soluble vitamins such as vitamin C are more likely to be lost by slowly heating up vegetables in cold water than if put in water that is already boiling.

Boiling and steaming cause only modest loss while inactivating some toxins and increasing the absorption of some nutrients.

Pressure cooking and microwave cooking retain most nutrients.

When animal fats or poly-unsaturated fats are over heated they form cholesterol oxidation products (trans-fats) which damage the arteries and harm health.

Avoid excess frying especially deep fat frying

Avoid overheating or re-using oil.

Poly-unsaturated oils exposed to light and heat and stored for a long time also form cholesterol oxidation products.

Store oils in dark containers and keep in the fridge.

Cook with monounsaturates such as olive, peanut or rapeseed oil or saturated fat such as butter or coconut oil. These form much less oxidation products (trans-fats).

General Advice Summary

- Eat plenty of fruit, vegetables, nuts, seeds and seed sprouts.

- Eat raw or lightly cooked vegetables (for low GI carbohydrate, protein, essential fatty acids, vitamins, minerals, fibre and phytonutrients).

- Have food that is as fresh as possible. Vegetable garden, allotment or locally grown plants are ideal. Frozen vegetables are almost as good.

- If not frozen, food requires preservatives to give it a reasonable shelf life and all preservatives in excess seem to be bad for your health.

- Eat plenty of fish (protein, essential fatty acids, vitamins, minerals and phytonutrients).

- Eat wholemeal rather than white bread (fibre, essential fatty acids, vitamins, minerals and phytonutrients).

- Drink plenty of water. If possible filter tap water or have mineral water, (to avoid chlorine, toxins etc).

- Exercise and keep active.

- Avoid very concentrated sweet food (high GI sugars).

- Avoid excess fried food such as chips and crisps (trans-fats).

- Avoid excess of processed food such as biscuits and cakes (excess preservatives such as sugar and salt, excess trans-fats).

- Avoid excess of dairy products such as cow's milk, cheese and butter (excess protein, excess saturated fat, excess calcium, low magnesium, excess hormones).

- Avoid excess meat especially if the animal is not grass fed and if it is from larger animals such as cows (excess protein, excess saturated fat, excess hormones).

- Avoid too many eggs (excess protein, excess saturated fat, excess hormones).

- Avoid excess salt.

- To lose weight: eat less. exercise more.

Essential nutrients: most commonly deficient					
Basic	Fats	Amino acids	Minerals	Vitamins	Phyto-nutrients
Oxygen	Linoleic acid (Omega 6)	Histidine	Calcium	A	**Flavonoids**
Light	**Linolenic acid (Omega 3)**	Isoleucine	**Chromium**	B1-thiamine	**Carotenoids**
Water		Leucine	Cobalt	B2-riboflavin	**Polyphenols**
Fibre		Lysine	Copper	**B3-niacin**	**Allyl sulphides**
Carbo-hydrate		Methionine	**Fluorine**	**B5-choline**	**Indoles**
		Pheny-lalanine	Iron	**B6-pyridoxine**	**Terpenes**
		Threonine	**Iodine**	**B-12**	**Protease inhibitors**
		Tryptophan	**Magnesium**	**Folic acid**	**Isoflavones**
		Valine	Manganese	Biotin	**Saponins**
			Moly-bdenum	**C-ascorbic acid**	**Lutein**
			Phosphorus	D	**Lycopene etc**
			Potassium	E	
			Selenium	K	
			Silicon		
			Sodium		
			Sulphur		
			Zinc		
			? Lithium		

Essential nutrients: most commonly excessive					
Basic	Fats	Amino acids	Minerals	Vitamins	Phyto-nutrients
Oxygen	**Linoleic acid (Omega 6)**	Histidine	**Calcium**	**A**	Flavonoids
Light	Linolenic acid (Omega 3)	Isoleucine	Chromium	B1-thiamine	Carotenoids
Water		Leucine	Cobalt	B2-riboflavin	Polyphenols
Fibre		Lysine	**Copper**	B3-niacin	Allyl sulphides
Carbo-hydrate		**Methionine**	Fluorine	B5-choline	Indoles
		Pheny-lalanine	Iron	B6-pyridoxine	Terpenes
		Threonine	Iodine	B-12	Protease inhibitors
		Tryptophan	Magnesium	Folic acid	Isoflavones
		Valine	Manganese	Biotin	Saponins
			Moly-bdenum	C-ascorbic acid	Lutein
			Phosphorus	D	Lycopene etc
			Potassium	E	
			Selenium	K	
			Silicon		
			Sodium		
			Sulphur		
			Zinc		
			? Lithium		

Good sources of:

Vitamins

Vitamin A: Animal products especially organs such as liver. Fish and fish oil, dairy products (milk, butter, cheese) and eggs, carrots, peppers, green vegetables.

Vitamin B: Wholegrain cereals and bread, nuts and seeds, beans, peas, meat , dairy products, eggs.

Vitamin B12: Liver, kidney, shellfish, fish, meat, soya beans. egg yolk.

Folic acid: Green leafy vegetables, beans, peas.

Vitamin C: Fruit and Vegetables.

Vitamin D: Animal and fish products, dairy products and eggs. Sunshine.

Vitamin E: Meat and fish, olive oil, avocado, eggs, dairy, seeds and nuts, wholegrain cereal and bread.

Vitamin K: Cauliflower, brussel sprouts, green leafy vegetables beans, potato, oily fish.

Essential fatty acids

Omega-3 (Linolenic acid): Oily fish, flax seeds, walnuts, green leafy vegetables, meat and eggs if animals fed on grass.

Omega-6 (Linoleic acid):   All nuts and seeds, especially corn, sesame and sunflower.

Good sources of:

Minerals

Boron: Fruits and vegetables.

Calcium: Green leafy vegetables beans and seeds, dairy products, fish.

Chromium: Wholegrain cereal and bread, beer, seafood, potatoes, eggs, chicken.

Iron: Dark meat. Beans, nuts and seeds, dates.

Magnesium: Wholegrain cereals and bread, green leafy vegetables, nuts, beans, peas, potato skin, raisins, garlic, crabs.

Manganese: Berries, beans, pineapple, chocolate.

Molybdenum: Tomatoes, wholegrain cereals and bread, beans, meat.

Phosphorus: Meat, dairy products, fruit and vegetables.

Potassium: Fruit and vegetables.

Selenium: Fish and seafood, wholegrain cereals and bread, liver, chicken, mushrooms, cabbage,

Sodium: Seafood, processed meat and dairy foods.

Sulphur: Fish, eggs, onions, garlic, cabbage.

Zinc: Fish and seafood, meat, egg yolk, wholegrain cereal and bread, nuts, peas, beans.

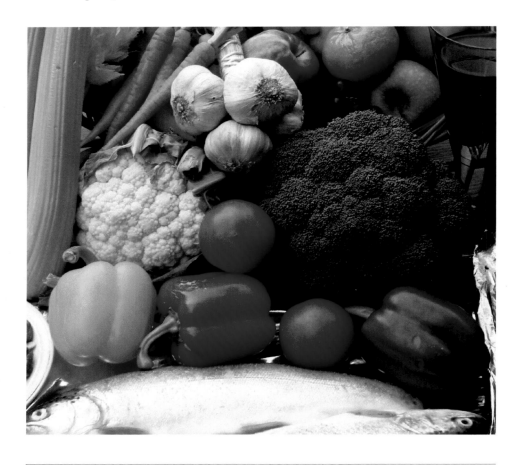

Main References

The New Optimum Nutrition Bible – Patrick Holford

Optimum Nutrition for the Mind – Patrick Holford.

Food is Better Medicine than Drugs – Patrick Holford & Jerome Burne.

Health Defence – Dr Paul Clayton.

Eating for Better Health – Professor Jane Plant and Gill Tidey.

Eating Well for Optimum Health – Dr Andrew Weil

Health Hazards of a Western Diet – George Stanton.

50 Ways to a Healthy Heart – Prof. Christiaan Barnard.

The Greek Doctors Diet – Dr. Fedon Alexander Lindberg.

Super Foods – Steven Pratt & Kathy Matthews

Cretan Cooking – Maria & Nikos Psilakis.

Plant based nutrition and health – Stephen Walsh.

The Great Cholesterol Con – Dr Malcolm Kendrick

Not another Guide to stress in General Practice – Dr. David Haslam.

Nutrition for Dummies – Nigel Denby, Sue Baic, Carol Ann Rinzler.

The Food Doctor – Ian Marber, Vicki Edgson.

Thorsons complete guide to Vitamins and Minerals – Leonard Mervyn

Vitamins & Minerals – Karen Sullivan.

Fundamentals of Clinical Nutrition –Sarah Morgan, Roland Weinser.

Nutrition and its Disorders – Donald McLaren.

Reader's Digest –*Guide to Vitamins, Minerals and Supplements.*

Reader's Digest – *Foods that harm, Foods that heal.*

Why you don't need Meat – Peter Cox

What are you Eating – Isabel Skypala.

Human Nutrition – Mary E. Barasi

Fast food Nation – Eric Schlosser.

Numerous articles, mainly in *The BMJ, GP, The Times* and *Sunday Times*.

Numerous articles, from the internet.